Make Up Your Face

Heather Card

Published in 2022 by Discover Your Bounce Publishing

www.discoveryourbouncepublishing.com

Copyright © Discover Your Bounce Publishing

ISBN 978-1-914428-05-0

Page design and typesetting by Discover Your Bounce
Publishing

DEDICATION

Dedicated to my distracting son Charlie (who was 9
months old at the beginning of this project) who was
absolutely no help when I was writing this book!

ACKNOWLEDGMENTS

Thank you to the Discover Your Bounce publishing team for making my dream of writing a makeup book come true. Thank you to my darling husband for sitting with me late into the night whilst I wrote this book, and to Rachel for the most beautiful illustrations and Mark for the fantastic design for the book cover.

CONTENTS

INTRODUCTION/HOW TO READ THIS BOOK

This book started life as a two-page handout I created to accompany my private makeup lessons. After starting to write about how to choose suitable foundation shades, tones, types and finishes, eight pages later I realised I still had lots more information and advice to give and Make Up Your Face was born.

After 8 years of managing and teaching makeup courses at 'Outstanding' colleges across the South West and over 10 years of freelance experience, to say I have a lot of resources is an understatement. Developing, managing and teaching BTEC HND, VRQ and NVQ courses gave me the perfect opportunity to produce my own makeup resources for my students to learn from.

The style this book is written in is designed to help the every-day makeup wearer like yourself to be able to choose suitable products, techniques and colours to best flatter and complement you, by first understanding the why and then the how. I have set out this book into the sections of the face thus if you want to learn about eye makeup you can go directly to the Eyes chapter and learn all about eye shapes, colours, products and application tools and techniques.

Throughout this book you can easily find personalised chapters and sections, so that you can read the chapters that you feel are more relevant to you although I do hope you will read it cover to cover. I have provided in-depth theory, tips and techniques and recommendations used for creating beautifully applied makeup to suit all occasions.

Makeup is subjective, it is an art. These are guidelines from a professional, they should not be seen as rules. I want you to feel beautiful and confident wearing your makeup.

Throughout this book I have chosen not to mention any brands in particular as I don't want to be seen to be affiliated with any brand over another. I use a wide variety of brands in my own makeup bag ranging from high-end, premium products to the more common high-street brands.

Without further ado, let's Make Up Your Face.

1. WAKE UP MAKEUP REGIME

1. Cleanse

If you only do three things for your skincare regime, make sure those are cleansing, exfoliating and moisturising.

Remove all your makeup at the end of the day and apply cleanser to the face before using any other skin or makeup product to remove any excess makeup, dirt, oil and pollutants from the skin.

2. Exfoliate

Exfoliate two to three times a week. Try not to exfoliate too often if you have dry or sensitive skin and try to use a gentler exfoliant to prevent causing any irritation to the skin. Mature skin types are better off exfoliating just twice a week.

If you wake up and your complexion is not glowing, you are better off exfoliating in the morning. Likewise, daily makeup wearers are better off exfoliating at night to remove any leftover or excess products left behind after cleansing the skin.

3. Moisturise

Moisturise your skin before applying your primer. It is best to use circular motions to apply your moisturiser to your face and don't forget your décolletage and neck as this is where we can show our age the most. When using your products, you need to make sure that you are lifting the face and not dragging it down, we want to fight against gravity's effect on our skin by lifting.

Apply a lip balm to your lips and let it soak in whilst you get on with the rest of your makeup.

4. Prime

Apply your choice of primer, using about a kidney bean size amount, and apply liberally all over the face, lips and eyes.

Choose a primer suitable for your skin type and don't be afraid to use a combination of different primers.

5. Eye Makeup

It is always good to prime the eyelids. You can use concealer to do this or an eyelid primer but make sure it sets before you apply any eye makeup, to prevent it from creasing. You can use a neutral tone shadow or translucent powder to set, then apply your choice of eye makeup, such as eyeliner, etc. Don't forget to highlight the inner corner of the eye to help open up and awaken your eyes.

6. Colour Correction

I like to colour correct before I apply foundation, or I will mix a colour corrector into my foundation; it all depends on what needs correcting to decide on the best course of action.

7. Foundation

Apply your suitable choice of foundation to the face.

Start in the centre of the face and blend outwards for a natural result. Be sure to apply using downward strokes to prevent the downy hairs from lifting and being accentuated with the product.

8. Concealer, Colour Correction

Apply your concealer after foundation; you will find you will need to use a lot less this way. Then you only need to apply concealer to any areas you may require slightly more coverage.

9. Contouring and Highlighting

Apply your choice of contouring product. If it is cream, make sure you set it with translucent powder before applying any powder blush or illuminator to the skin, to prevent the makeup from going patchy.

10. Blush

Ensure you set your base if you are going to be using a powder blush. If you are using a wax or cream formula, then you do not need to set your base before applying these products as they will look the most natural when the product is melted into the skin.

Make sure you place your blusher in the correct position to suit your face shape.

11. Setting Your Makeup

Set your base with translucent powder or pressed powder. Spray a setting spray over the entire face to prolong the longevity of your makeup.

12. Brows

Measure, shape and define your brow; use concealer in a paler shade under the brow's arch to help elevate the face.

13. Mascara

Apply your mascara choice to the roots of your lashes and give the mascara wand a wiggle as you lift through the lashes to ensure the product coats every lash. This will provide volume and length.

I like to apply a coat of mascara to my lashes before I apply false lashes, and I will curl them too however, it can cause the lashes to lift significantly, causing problems trying to fit strip lashes.

14. False Lashes

Measure your lashes and cut the length of the lash strip from the outer corner. Apply glue to the strip lash and allow the glue to go tacky. Whilst looking down into a mirror (so your eyes are not closed, making it easier to stick your lashes on) apply your lashes to your natural lash line and using your index finger and thumb, press the strip lashes and natural lashes together. Finally, apply a coat of mascara to blend the lashes together for a more natural result. A great tip is to apply eyeliner to the upper waterline into the inner corner of the eye, this will help your false lashes seamlessly blend into your natural lash line.

2. MAKEUP LIFE EXPECTANCY

We all know that makeup does not last forever, especially if we use it every day, but did you know that all your makeup has a shelf life? A life expectancy. Using out of date products can expose you to harmful toxins and bacteria that could cause serious health problems. That is why I am going to tell you exactly how often you should be replenishing your makeup and to give you some hints and tips to prolong the longevity of your makeup.

The life expectancy of any makeup product can be affected by the way it is used and stored. All makeup expires eventually, usually within 2 to 3 years as a general rule. Still, every cosmetic is different and usually has an expiry date stamped on the package (PAO which stands for 'Period after opening'), i.e. (on the product label you will see a small picture of an opened tub with a number and an M next to it) This indicates how many months you have until it expires.

This is all well and good if you remember which month you purchased it in. Still, suppose you are not an avid makeup wearer and the product is put into a makeup bag, never to be seen again. In that case, you may find when you do come to use it that it may be past its best. Or, if you are like me and have lots of cosmetics in rotation, it is hard to take stock of expiry dates. So, I always like to label my products when I get them with a number that represents the month and year I purchased them.

Preservatives in makeup will eventually break down; formulas will separate or spoil. Natural products may go off even sooner due to the lack of preservatives used in their manufacturing.
If you use your makeup products regularly, you should have no problem using them up before their expiry date.

Heat and humidity are not suitable for makeup and

may cause the products to oxidise, melt, separate or change colour, and they will not perform to the optimal capacity.

I recommend storing your makeup in a dry, cool area like a vanity case, draw or cupboard. I would refrain from keeping your makeup in a humid bathroom or on a hot windowsill.

Foundation and Concealer: 18-24 Months

Ideally, your foundation and concealer should last between 18 and 24 months but always follow the manufacturer's guidelines (PAO).

Always apply your foundation with freshly washed hands, clean brushes and try to decant the product before using it to prevent introducing bacteria into your foundation. Powder foundations will last considerably longer, up to 2 years, before they need replacing.

Powder Products: 12-24 Months

Yes, powder products do expire. Although they contain no liquid to harbour bacteria, they can be affected by our natural skin oils and particles of other cream cosmetics. Eyeshadow and blush should last between 12 and 24 months but always follow the manufacturer's guidelines (PAO).

To prolong the life expectancy of your powder products, make sure you are using a clean, dry brush every time to apply your blush or eyeshadow. Also, always wait for your base to be dry or set before applying a powder product. Do not be tempted to use a wet foundation brush to apply your power product, as the oils in the foundation can interfere with the powder, causing them to oxidise and become unusable.

Always make sure the lid is tightly fastened after every use.

Lipstick and Gloss: 18-24 Months

We all have that favourite colour lippy that we keep for decades, but did you know that lipstick should really only be kept and used for up to 2 years? This is because lipstick will start to dry out and gloss will turn gloopy as it is exposed to oxygen. In addition, lipsticks often contain lots of oils and preservatives, preventing the build-up of bacteria; however, after about a year, these will start to break down. Always follow the manufacturer's POA.

To prolong the longevity of your lipstick, try decanting some of the product and use a lip brush to apply; this will prevent introducing any bacteria onto the lipstick. If you develop a cold sore or anything infectious around the mouth, then I recommend that you throw away your lipstick as the likelihood is that it is already contaminated and you don't want to reintroduce the bacteria back onto your face.

Try to store your lippy in a cool, dry place like a vanity case or drawer as keeping it in a humid bathroom can cause the pigments to eventually break down and separate. You also don't want to store your favourite lippy in heat or humidity as this will soften the formula causing it to be challenging to apply accurately, and it could cause the lipstick to snap off inside the applicator which is so annoying.

If your lipstick has beads of moisture on its surface, smells, or has turned chalky, it is time to replace it.

Lipliners and Eyeliners: 3 Months-3 Years

Liquid eyeliner has the same shelf life as mascara because it has the same bacteria prone formula and tubular packaging.

To help your liquid liner last longer, try cleaning the applicator after every use, before storing it away.

Eyeliner and lipliner pencils have a longer shelf life of three years as they can be sharpened between each application, therefore removing any bacteria that may have previously been picked up.

Make sure you clean your sharpener too with IPA (isopropyl alcohol or rubbing alcohol) to prevent it from harbouring any germs and transferring them onto your pencil liners.

Always follow the individual product POA.

Mascaras: 3-6 Months

If worn every day, then believe it not, it needs replacing every 3months; if you use it occasionally, then every 6 months will suffice. Mascara is a significant harbourer of bacteria. Not only is the wet consistency an ideal breeding ground for bugs, but the fact that the applicator touches the lashes, that contain naturally occurring germs, and is then put back into the tube contributes to its short shelf life.

Mascara, if kept for a long time, will not only turn gloopy and dry out with exposure to air, it can also harbour some sinister bugs like staph.

As a professional makeup artist, I always use disposable mascara wands to prevent introducing any bacteria into my mascara tube. I use my mascara so often I replace it every 6 months anyway.

I recommend not pumping the mascara wand in and out of the tube, this introduces air into the tube and causes the formula to dry out. If your mascara has gone a little sticky, try adding a couple of drops of baby oil and you should be good to go.

Always adhere to the manufacturer's guideline POA.
The POA is averaged, and if you were to use the product after the expiry date, you are likely to be okay.

If you have an eye infection or anything contagious like a cold sore or a skin infection, etc, I strongly recommend throwing away your makeup and replacing it to prevent reintroducing the infection back onto the skin or anywhere else.

If you find that you are suffering from unexplained break-outs, then try washing your makeup brushes more often. Check the expiry dates on your makeup and throw away any out of date makeup or anything that smells or has separated (within reason; it may just require a shake). Any pressed powders with a greyish film over them or anything that is discoloured, you are better off throwing out and replacing. Your skin will thank you for it later, and it really can make a big difference.

If you find a product that has dried up, or perhaps you want a powder colour to be more vivid, please do not be tempted to lick your brush or introduce any saliva into the product, as this will only introduce bacteria into your makeup. Instead, try adding a little bit of baby oil to reinvigorate a mascara or eyeliner, and use a setting spray or clean water to wet your brush to make your colours more vivid.

3. HOW TO CLEAN YOUR MAKEUP BRUSHES AND SPONGES

Cleaning your brushes should be an essential part of anyone's makeup regime. Maintaining healthy, clean and sanitised brushes is a must if you want to get the best out of your makeup application at home.
As a minimum, brushes should be cleaned every 2 weeks.

Sponges and beauty blenders are major harbourers of bacteria and should ideally be washed after every use.
Run the sponge under warm water until the water runs clear for a quick rinse, or try using antibacterial dish soap. Emulsify in a bit of water in your hand and

then run under a tap until the water runs clear and squeeze out any suds, whilst being careful not to rip your beauty blender, then place it on a dry paper towel to dry.

Never leave your brushes to soak, whether it's an IPA or soap water solution, as this can cause the glue holding your brush together to disintegrate and cause bristles to loosen and fall out. When drying your brushes, always ensure that they are facing down so water cannot run up your handle and eventually cause damage to the handle and the glue.

IPA Cleaning Method

Ingredients you will need:

- IPA (isopropyl alcohol) 80%.
- A glass jar or spray bottle.
- Paper towels.
- Tea towel or hand towel.

I clean my kit brushes after every client as I have to ensure no bugs or germs are left on my brushes. I like to use IPA isopropyl alcohol, which is 90% alcohol, to sanitise and clean my brushes. Also, IPA air dries, so it is excellent if you want to use your brushes almost immediately after washing them.

I recommend using a small glass tumbler or jar to put the IPA into as some plastics will melt, either instantly or over time.

You only need your IPA to be as deep as your brush bristle because it evaporates so you don't want to fill up a whole glass and end up wasting it. Make sure you replace the IPA after every few brushes to ensure you are using clean IPA to remove dirt from your brushes and not just washing grime and germs back into your brushes.

You can dip your brush in IPA, then swirl it onto a paper towel and repeat until clean. Or you can put IPA in a water spray bottle (make sure it is labelled and kept out of reach of children), and spray it directly onto the brush bristles and repeat the process until the paper towel comes up clean. Using a spray is a good method when you are on the go if you want to use the brush again immediately after, as the brush is often not as wet as it would be if you were to dunk it.

Antibacterial Washing Up Liquid Cleaning Method

Ingredients you will need:

- Antibacterial washing up liquid.
- Colander.
- Bowl of warm water or sink.
- Paper towels.
- Tea towel or hand towel.

My new favourite way to clean my own personal brushes is to use antibacterial washing up liquid, warm water and a colander. You read that correctly, a colander – the thing you drain your veg in – makes the perfect tool for cleaning makeup brushes!

I put the washing up liquid into the bottom of the colander and place the colander into a washing up bowl of warm water. I then dip my brushes into the antibacterial liquid and use the holes of the colander to help clean right to the root of the brush by rubbing the brush across them using a stirring action. I dip my brush into the water and then rinse it under the tap to clean out the soap. The brushes are left to dry on a tea towel or small towel or I hang them over the edge of the sink to prevent them from becoming misshapen.

You can really see the dirt coming out with this method, so make sure you change the water often to prevent harbouring germs and bacteria in your brushes.

Baby Shampoo Cleaning Method

Ingredients you will need:

- Baby shampoo or olive oil.
- Washbowl/colander.
- Paper towels.
- Tea towel or hand towel.

Using baby shampoo is another good product to clean your brushes with. It is not antibacterial, so some bacteria may still be present, lurking somewhere in your brushes but using shampoo does keep the quality of the bristle soft and your brushes smelling great.

Unfortunately, brushes do not last forever and

experts say to replace them every 3-4 months, but if you look after your brushes, they will look after you and can and will last a lot longer. However, if they do start to shed, I recommend getting rid of them, as it will only worsen and affect your makeup application.

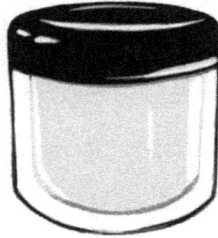

4. SKINCARE

When deciding which foundation you are going to use, you first need to determine your skin type to ensure your choice of foundation is compatible with your skin and its needs. You don't want to starve dry skin of moisture or over saturate an oily skin with more oil as this may cause additional issues. The best way to decide on your skin type is to look at your skin in natural light when your skin is free from all grease, oil and dirt.

SKIN TYPES

Normal skin	• Normal skin is not too dry and not too oily • No or few imperfections • No severe sensitivity • Barely visible pores • A naturally radiant complexion
Sensitive skin	• Sensitive skin can show up as redness • Itching • Burning • Dry • It can be affected by products used on the skin, weather and environment
Combination skin	• A combination skin type can be dry or normal in some areas and oily in others, such as the T-zone (nose, forehead and chin)

	• Many people have combination skin, which may benefit from slightly different types of skincare in each area • Overly dilated pores • Blackheads • Shiny skin
Oily skin	• Oily skin can produce enlarged pores • Dull or shiny, thick complexion • Blackheads, pimples and/or other blemishes • Oiliness can change depending upon the time of year or the weather
Dry skin	• Dry skin has almost invisible pores • Dull, rough complexion • Red patches • Less elasticity • More visible lines

SKIN PREP: CLEANSE, TONE AND MOISTURISE

You have now identified your skin type. Next, your skin needs to be prepared for the makeup application. It is always best to work with a clean canvas when applying makeup as any grease, dirt or patchy skin will affect your overall makeup application. Your makeup can only be as good as your skin!

Cleanse

1. Remove all eye makeup using a cotton wool pad and eye makeup remover. I personally love micellar water as I find it removes even the toughest of makeup, such as waterproof eyeliner and mascara. Ensure you wipe away from the eye and make sure you use a new cotton pad for each eye.

2. When removing your mascara, I always like to fold a cotton pad in half and place it under the top lashes with a closed eye and use another cotton pad or bud with the eye

makeup remover to wipe away the mascara gently; never scrub your eye as you may cause your lashes to break off or fall out.

3. Remove lipstick using the same remover and apply a lip balm to soften the lips whilst applying the rest of the makeup.

4. There are many varieties of cleansers available on the market, so make sure you use the right one for your skin type. Apply your chosen cleanser to the face and neck using clean hands or a cotton pad using upward strokes across the neck and outward strokes across the jawline. Use small circular motions across the T-zone starting on the chin, circle across the cheeks and finish at the temples.

5. Remove the cleanser from the skin with dampened cotton pads using two hands. Follow the same pattern as applying to remove the cleanser and repeat until your cotton pads are coming off the face clean. It may take a couple of passes across the face to remove all the skin's grease and dirt.

Tone

6. Use a cotton pad saturated in toner and sweep in circular motions gently across the face and neck, avoiding the eye area.

7. If you have combination skin, you may wish to apply toner to the oiliest area of the face, usually the T-zone and around the sides of the nose.

Moisturise

8. You can use clean hands or a large flat brush to apply your moisturiser. Apply a ten pence size piece into the palm of your hands and apply it to the face, avoiding the delicate eye area. Use circular motions across the face and upward strokes on the jawline and neck.

9. If you have an oily skin type, I suggest using a water-based moisturiser to prevent oversaturating your skin with excess oil.

10. If you have combination skin, you may wish to apply moisturiser to the dry areas of the face to give those areas added hydration.

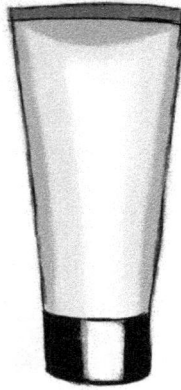

5. PRIMERS

Primer is simple. It's exactly what its name implies: a product that's applied after your skin care routine, before your makeup application, to create an ideal canvas to hold onto whatever makeup comes afterward, such as foundation, tinted moisturiser or concealer.

Primer is one of the more mysterious and puzzling base products on the market. There is such a vast array of different primer options available that all claim to do something different, e.g. hydrating, mattifying, blurring or luminating. It can be very confusing to figure out which type of primer will work best for you.

There are different formulations of primers, just like foundations, containing different ingredients, including hyaluronic acid that boosts hydration, a SPF that softens the appearance of pores, Salicylic acid to mattify the complexion, some primers contain antioxidants like vitamin A, C and E, and others are the traditional silicone-based primer that smooths and blurs.

Whilst some primers work to reduce the size of visible pores, add hydration, brighten complexion or colour correct, others help minimise the appearance of fine lines and wrinkles, target acne and can even give a temporary face-lift. Primers are best known for their mattifying qualities and prolonging the makeup to stop it from slipping or caking on the skin.

As with a foundation or concealer, you want to choose a primer that is suited to your skin type and that will work well with your choice of foundation product, e.g. A primer that is mostly silicone-based will cause a foundation that is mostly water to slide off the skin regardless of how much you try to set it.

Do I Need a Primer?

I don't believe there is a short answer here as it's about evaluating any issues you may have with your skin and how happy you are with your overall face-makeup look, feel and finish.

Is there something missing? Maybe you want more of a youthful glow or perhaps you feel too shiny. A primer could be precisely what you need to address these issues.

When I am designing and choosing suitable products to use on my clients, these are the things that I think about and they should be something you think about when deciding if you want or need to use a primer.

- Do you feel conscious about the size of your pores?
- Do you need an extra step to help mattify your skin?
- Do you need a hydration boost?
- Do you need a primer with anti-ageing properties?

- Do you need an extra step to even your complexion out?

Application of Face Primer

- Use clean fingers to apply primer. I find this gives a seamless finish, as a makeup brush can just drag the primer around. If you do not fancy using your fingers then use a slightly damp beauty blender to blend the product into the skin.

- Less is more when it comes to primer, a 10 pence piece size is a sufficient amount to apply to the entire face. Apply lightly and sparingly.

- Base the amount of primer you use on your skin type, for example, someone with a dry skin can use more primer than someone with an oily skin because the skin will absorb it faster. However, someone with an oily skin should refrain from oversaturating their skin with primer as it will just sit on the surface of the skin instead of being absorbed and is likely to disrupt the makeup application.

- Use a separate eye primer as they have slightly different ingredients that are designed for use on the delicate eye area.

- Make sure you wait at least a minute before applying any other makeup product over the top of your primer to avoid disrupting the makeup.

I always believe less is more, especially when it comes to preparing the skin for the application of makeup. I have seen so many YouTubers doing demonstrations where they apply a primer, shimmer oil, colour corrector, concealer and then a full coverage foundation and pressed powder. I am sorry but no amount of blending is ever going to truly conceal the amount of product that will still be evident on the surface of the skin in these cases. It is just not necessary. You will achieve a much more natural look by applying less product.

Eye Primer

There are lots of eye primers on the market but they all pretty much do the same job. They even out the colour of the eyelid by covering any discolouration, redness or veins and they remove any oil from the skin. They can add shimmer or be matte in nature but all primers aid in the smooth application of eyeshadow, intensify eyeshadow colours and prevent the eyeshadow from creasing as well as improving the longevity of the eye makeup.

Eye primer is applied to the eyelid and lower eye lash area and blended into the skin prior to the application of eyeshadow.

Lash/Mascara Primer

Lash primer tends to be colourless and comes in packaging that very much looks like clear mascara. It is often applied with the mascara wand and is used to thicken or lengthen the natural lashes before the application of mascara. There are varieties that can also help the lashes to grow.

Lip Primer

Lip primers are intended to smooth the lip and to help with the adhesion and longevity of lipliner, lipstick and gloss. It also prevents the lipstick from "feathering", where the lipstick product sits in the fine lines around the lips and smears, although a lipliner can help with this and so will a primer applied to the lip before any other lip products are applied.

Not all makeup artists will agree that you must wear primer every time you put on your makeup. I don't always apply primers to all my clients; as long as I am happy that I have prepared the skin thoroughly and it is well hydrated, I am happy to continue primer free. I think it is more about personal choice, your skin type and whether you are happy with your makeup finish without a primer.

As I work with lots of different clients with different skin types and conditions, I like to stock a variety of different primers in my kit. These include: Gosh primer, which is like silk when it is applied, especially for a cheaper high street brand, and NYX pore filler and E.L.F primers are good as they are designed and packaged for different issues such as hydration, pore moisturise, mattifying, radiance, etc. so I have a few of these products in my kit.

Sometimes I still feel like something is needed between the skin and the foundation so I like to use Embryolisse Lait-Crème. A firm favourite amongst makeup artists, it's a vitamin and antioxidant enriched moisturiser that is slightly thick, is designed for dry skin and gives a lovely soft satin finish to the skin.

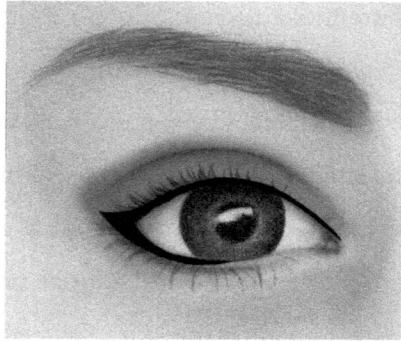

6. EYES

EYESHADOW

There are many different types of eyeshadow products available on the market and they all create different effects and finishes. An eyeshadow is not just available in a powder finish, you can also get creams, gels, pigment powders and foil finishes that all give dramatically different looks.

With so many eyeshadows available on the market, it is hard to decide not only what colour to choose but which brand, type and finish would suit you best and it can be overwhelming to make a choice.

I am hopefully going to give you all the information you need so you can confidently choose the right product type and colours to suit you, your eyes and desired look.

Whether you are looking for something subtle and natural or you want to create a statement with a bright or bold eye look then there is a perfect eyeshadow for you.

There are seven main types of eyeshadow on the market, the most common is made of powder, also known as pressed powder, and it normally comes in a palette format. Then there is liquid, cream, stick or crayon and pigments.

As with any makeup, there is not a one-size-fits-all approach when it comes to eye makeup. There are some valid uses for the different types of eyeshadow and I am here to tell you about them and how to successfully and effectively choose the most suitable product that's right for you and helps you create your desired look.

That being said I am not trying to burst anyone's creativity and I want you to feel beautiful and confident in your own skin, so you should use whatever product you like. I am only giving some helpful guidelines for you to make the best choice if you are looking to wake up your makeup.

Prep and Prime

Priming the eye is so important if you want your eye makeup to last throughout the day and if you want your makeup colours to pop.

Eye primer works just like a facial primer; it prepares the eye for makeup, giving you a smooth canvas to work on and something for the product to cling too, prolonging its staying power.

You need to prep your eye area before applying any primers or concealers. I recommend applying an eye cream to help soften and moisturise the eye area to minimise fine lines, reduce dark circles and plump up the skin. Do not apply directly to the eyelid or too close to the lower lashes, as the product is likely to travel when it warms up with your body heat, potentially causing discomfort and pain if it was to make contact with your eye.

When it comes to priming your eye there is a vast

variety of products available to you, but they all basically do the same thing. They neutralise the eye area – remove any redness, blue tones, discolouration and pigmentation – whilst providing a neutral tone to work on top of. This helps eyeshadow colours to stay vivid. The primer will remove the natural oils from the eyelid ensuring that your makeup will be less likely to crease, smudge and transfer and this will prolong its staying power too.

You could buy an eye primer product but you can also use your skin tone concealer that you likely already have as part of your makeup bag. Sweep your concealer all over your entire lid and brow bone, blend in by lightly patting with a ring finger and set with a translucent powder or skin tone eyeshadow powder.

I recommend priming or neutralising your eyes each time before applying any other eye makeup products to make your look fresh, durable and to help make those colours pop.

Powder

Powder is the most common types of eyeshadow, the

one everyone is familiar with and would have seen across multiple brands or Christmas box sets.

Powder eyeshadows are condensed in containers, often in a palette format, providing you with a wide choice of colours and finishes in matte, satin and shimmer.

Some brands, when creating their palettes, set them out to be easy to use as they provide you with all the shades you need to create your eye makeup look. These are often made up of:

Base – this shade can be applied to the entire eyelid from lashes to brow and can be used to set primer.

Highlight – this shade can be used under the brow bone, applied to the inner corner of the eye and the eye lid, and it can be used on its own or blended with a darker shade.

Transition – this shade is used to define the natural crease. It can add dimension to the eye, minimise a hooded eye, add depth to a mono-lid and it can be used to help blend the light and dark shades together without muddying the effect.

Definition – th_s is a darker shade used to add definition across the lash lines, smoke out the outer corner and it can be used as an eyeliner or on its own to create a smoky eye look.

Some brands may only provide you with the choice of two or three tones of dark and light eyeshadows whilst others may provide you with a whole host of rainbow colours for you to be able to create your own funky designs. Palettes come in a variety of different sizes and finishes of matte, shimmery and satin. You can get palettes that are either entirely in one colour spectrum, such as pink, gold, blues, etc., or one finish, such as matte neutral tones, or they can provide you with a tailored mix of matte and shimmer shades and are often set out in a way that is easy to follow.

Powder eyeshadow is a great place to start for beginners as they are reasonably inexpensive depending on what brand you buy. They are easy to use and can be applied with a makeup brush or even a finger and they are very forgiving as they can easily be blended out and built up to intensify the colours.

I would recommend having a palette that gives you the option of both matte and shimmery shades so you can experiment with creating different looks in different finishes; matte for every day or period looks. Satin is also suitable to wear every day but also for weddings and evenings, and the shimmer glittery shades are great for creating dramatic evening looks. You can mix and match the finishes or use them separately, it is entirely up to you.

It is recommended in the industry that shimmery finishes are not suitable for mature eyes as the shine can highlight fine lines and wrinkles but I disagree. I often use satin shades on my mature clients as I find matte shades can often look ageing. It all depends on your desired look and makeup goals.

When applying your eyeshadow I recommend using a flat eyeshadow brush to gently pat on and deposit the colour onto the eye lid and using a soft, fluffy crease brush for any blending, ensuring you do not drag or pull on the delicate skin on and around the eye.

Baked Powder

What is the difference between an eyeshadow powder and a baked powder? Well, the baked powder isn't actually a pressed powder at all, it is a cream formula that has been baked slowly to remove the moisture, oils, etc, producing a beautifully soft, marbled, velvety powder. Baked powder is a fairly new concept to the industry and is available in a variety of products including blushers, bronzers and highlighters.

With its ultra-smooth, illuminating finish, that is easily blended and built-up quality, it's the ideal product for creating long-lasting eye looks.

Baked powder can be applied both wet and dry. If you dampen your brush with a little bit of setting spray or a spritz of water this will not only intensify the colour of the powder but it will also help it last much longer on the eyes.

Baked powder products often have a marbled appearance and give an illuminous finish giving a beautiful sheen to the skin without being too glittery or thick and I highly recommend purchasing a palette or two to go in your makeup kit.

Liquid

Liquid eyeshadows come in the same packaging as most lip gloss, in a sleek tube with a fluffy wand and, like powder eyeshadow, they are the perfect product for beginners as they are so easy to use. You simply swipe the wand over the lid or you can use a fine liner brush to create a beautiful bold eyeliner look.

Liquid eyeshadow, although it is easy to use, does dry very quickly so there is little room for error and not much blending time.

A lot like the cream formula, liquid shadows can crease so I do not recommend using them on a hot day or if you have particularly oily eyelids as the oil and heat can make the liquid move about and travel causing the shadow to crease more. I like to use liquid eyeshadows as a base for my pigments to cling to as it enhances their vibrancy and longevity.

Cream

Cream eyeshadows often come in small pots but can also be found in pans, tubes and stick form as well.

Cream products offer bold colours with a shimmery finish and are often long wearing but can be prone to creasing and transferring. I recommend priming the eye well before applying a cream shadow to prevent transfer and apply a powder or pigment over the top of the cream to prevent the product from sliding. I do not recommend wearing this formula in heat as it is likely to melt as it is not waterproof.

Cream shadows are easy to use and because of their consistency, they are blendable so you can mix two or more colours together for a bolder look.

I recommend applying a cream shadow with an eyeshadow brush/large shader brush to pack on the colour for a bolder result.

Foil (Foiling)

Foil eyeshadow is the cross between a cream and a baked powder and is often in a pan (palette) format or a tube.

Foil shadows are often metallic and glam and when applied right they can give a molten metal liquid look shine to your eyelids. The texture is wetter than a baked powder but not as runny as a liquid, it gives a beautiful smooth application and a rich payoff with its colour and longevity. This is the perfect product for any beginner to create a truly professional looking result with ease.

There are lots of foil eyeshadows available on the market, often as part of palettes alongside matte and other shimmery shades, but you can, in fact, create your own foil shadow using cream eyeshadow or even a powder shadow. Simply spritz a flat eyeshadow brush with a setting spray and dip the brush into the cream or powder and apply multiple layers to your eyelid, ideally above the iris or to the inner corner for a beautiful pop of glam.

You can also mix a metallic pigment or choice of shadow with a mixing medium, like primer or an eye base primer, to intensify the colour and prevent it from fading, smudging and creasing.

For a pre-made foil shadow, I recommend using a finger to apply this product as the heat from your hands softens the formula for a professional looking result.

Make sure, whether you use setting spray or a primer, that your brush is not too wet. It should just feel slightly damp, and try not to oversaturate your shadow mix otherwise you risk diluting the pigment and could end up with a runny mess.

Foil shadows can be used on their own or on top of other eyeshadow products and look great applied in the centre of the eyelid, inner corner or a sweep all over the eye will look amazing too. Make sure your eyelid is well primed before applying your choice of foil.

Stick and Crayon

If you are looking for something super easy to use, perhaps use on the go, then a crayon is perfect for you. You literally draw onto your eyelids with the pigmented crayon. It can also be applied to your lower lash line and the waterline without too much fuss and you can blend with a finger if you wish but you don't have to, you can just glide it on and go. Crayons typically consist of intense pigment and primer as part of their formula which gives them a staying power of up to 24 hours of wear.

This product is ideal for keeping in your handbag for touch ups throughout the day or to take your day makeup into the night.

Pigments

Pigment eyeshadows are similar to powder but they are a lot looser. The formula is finely milled and highly pigmented. They come in pots with twist-on lids and offer the most pigment out of all the eyeshadow products but due to their intense pigmentation and tendency to be messy, they do require lots of practice. I highly recommend doing your eye makeup first, then you can tidy up any fallout (when eyeshadow drops under the eye) or clean up any dodgy edges with your foundation and concealer.

I do not recommend this type of shadow for mature or dry skin as it is likely to accentuate your fine lines and wrinkles and dry out the skin further.

These are fantastic for their colour range and boldness. You will definitely need to prime your eyes before using this product for it to stick. Alternatively, try wetting your makeup brush (do not lick it) with a wipe or dip it in some setting spray before using it to apply your pigment. It will minimise the mess whilst enhancing the colour.

Glitter, Sequins and Gems

Sequins and gems are probably not for your everyday makeup wearer however, they are fantastic for clubs, gigs, shows and festivals.

Here are my top tips for applying your own embellishment to your makeup.

Application Tips for Applying Embellishment

- **Top tip:** never be tempted to apply craft glitter to your face and body. Yes, it is cheaper and probably easier to get hold of but it can be quite dangerous. Craft glitter is not cut rounded like cosmetic body glitter so if it was to go into the eye it could cause quite a bit of damage whereas the cosmetic glitter, although uncomfortable, is unlikely to cause long-term damage.

- When applying glitter, I like to mix two or three different sizes of glitter for an extra wow factor. Try using an ultra-fine glitter with a chunky glitter to give your makeup extra depth, vibrancy, shine and colour.

- Use a hard-set hair gel as a cheap alternative to glitter glue. Apply this to the area where the glitter will be added and then pat on your mix of textures.

- Use an eyelash glue for adding gems, fabric, sequins or beads, etc. Use tweezers to hold the sequin, dot a small amount of glue onto the back of the sequin and let it go tacky for a couple of seconds, then press it onto the skin to secure it in place.

- To remove, simply use an oily eye makeup remover, gently pat over the area and peel off any large pieces.

Cosmetic glitter can be applied to all areas of the face. There are special glues available for the lips and eyes, but I have found cheaper alternatives; if you use a cream eyeshadow base on your eyelids and pat the glitter onto this, then it dries and stays put just like a glue. If you apply a lip gloss to your lips then you can pat the glitter directly on top. It's worth noting that I have found that some glues can often be hard to remove at the end of an event.

EYELINER

There are three main types of eyeliner: pencil, gel and liquid. But which is best?

These eyeliners all have different qualities. Some are smudgeable and are great for creating a smoky eye, whilst others are inky, fast drying, really black and are great for creating a bold graphic statement.

Depending on your desired look and needs,

eyeliner comes in a variety of formulas and colours and can be applied to different areas of the eye and face and used to achieve different looks.

It is useful to know how you intend to use your eyeliner, what you hope to achieve and your application skills when choosing the most suitable product for you.

These are the three main types of eyeliner available on the market:

Pencil Eyeliner

Pencil liner is the most common form of eyeliner and comes in – you guessed it – pencil form. You can get all the colours of the rainbow too, so it is a very versatile product.

Easy to use and most formulas of pencil are blendable so perfect for creating sultry smoky eyes. The pencil liner can be applied to the top and bottom lash line and waterlines too, just make sure you are not trying to use a waterproof formula when applying eyeliner to your waterline as it won't work.

I recommend having a black, brown and cream

concealer colour liner in your makeup kit. The brown could be used for your brows too, the cream colour can be used as a lipliner, on the waterline to make your eyes look bigger and on the inner corner of the eye to awaken the eye.

Always make sure you sharpen your pencil between each use to remove any bacteria.

Rub your eyeliner pencil between the palms of your hand to help soften the formula for an easier application.

Kohl Pencil Eyeliner

Kohl eyeliner, like the pencil eyeliner, comes in a pencil form but it is more well-known for its creaminess and is much easier to smudge and blend, unlike a standard wax pencil liner, so it can be used to create smoky eyes without the drag.

Kohl eyeliner can be applied to the top and bottom lashes and the waterline, and because of its creamy formula it applies easily to the waterline without the drag of a wax formula and without the need to retrace your line, causing unwanted irritation to the eye.

If you wanted to create a smoky eye using just an eyeliner then I would recommend using a Kohl eyeliner, however because of its blend ability it does not last as long as an original pencil.

Gel Eyeliner

I am a bit of an advocate for gel liner as I use this formula a lot with my clients and on myself. I like it because, again, it is versatile with a wide choice of colours available. It is quite wet so I find it very easy to apply without drag and I can choose whichever brush I wish to apply it, which is often a thin angled brush or square-ended brush.

Gel liner can be used on the top and bottom lash lines and often on the waterline too as once the formula is applied and dries completely; it cannot be blended so it works well on the waterline as it won't transfer or smudge once dry.

A little trick to try when applying gel liner to your waterline is dipping a pencil liner in the gel liner as sometimes a brush or cotton bud can cause irritation to the eye.

You can blend it before it dries so you can create

both graphic lines, flicks and shapes or softer smudges and blends for smoky eyes.

Once dry it becomes waterproof due to its high wax content and therefore is perfect for everyday wear or perhaps when you need something long-lasting and durable for a special occasion.

Because this type of eyeliner is waterproof it needs to be removed with a good makeup remover and as always, I recommend using micellar water.

Liquid Eyeliner

There are two forms of liquid eyeliner: there is the type that looks similar to a felt tip pen and the other that looks like a mini nail varnish type bottle with its own brush applicator with a really long thin bristle.

I prefer to use separate makeup brushes to apply this type of liquid eyeliner as I find the thin brush included difficult to control.

The felt tip pen type is inky and you can literally draw with it on the eyelid so it is easy to use, but it can't be blended as it dries quickly. I would not recommend using this type of liner on the waterline due to its high alcohol content as it is likely to vapour and cause discomfort, and it won't dry.

Liquid eyeliner requires lots of practice with the application as it dries so quickly there is no room for error, however, it is still a great product for creating long-lasting wings, flicks and graphic lines and for avant-garde looks.

Eyeshadow Eyeliner

Although I said there are three main types of eyeliner, there is in fact a fourth type. You can create your own eyeliner using your choice of powder or cream eyeshadow or blush by simply applying it directly as a powder or mix your product with water, setting spray or a mixer to create a liquid form of colour that you can then use to paint onto the eyelid. This is not recommended for use on the waterline but it is suitable and safe to use on the top and bottom lash lines.

Now you have chosen your ideal eyeliner product, here are some top tips to help you apply your best liner.

Application Tips for Applying Your Eyeliner

Here are some hints, tips, tricks and hacks for applying your eyeliner but like all makeup it requires practice so just have fun creating your eyeliner looks, practice makes perfect.

- If you're just starting out applying eyeliner then I recommend using dots or dashes across the lash line and then connecting them instead of trying to apply your eyeliner all in one go and making mistakes.

- For extra stability when applying your eyeliner I recommend you sit down, plant an elbow on a flat surface and use your pinkie or the edge of your palm rested on your cheek to steady your hand for a neater application.

- Don't stretch the eye out with your fingers as this can distort your application. Try just looking down instead of completely closing your eye as this will help maximise your eyelid surface. Use a cotton bud and makeup remover to tidy up any mistakes. Concealer can also be used to help neaten up any lines.

- Use a pencil crease brush, also known as a smudger brush, to blend and smoke out an imperfect line.

- Use some black eyeshadow to help fill in and neaten a line or use it as a guide to follow for a precise liquid or gel liner application.

- If you don't like eyeliner on you, but you want your natural lashes to look fuller then try a tight line. This is when you apply liner to the top waterline underneath your lashes along the top lash line. I love using this technique when I do any eyeliner as sometimes skin can still be visible no matter how close you get to the lash line. This is a great technique I often use when I am creating a natural look or perhaps if I only have a few minutes to do my makeup in the morning, this gives me instant definition and thicker looking lashes.

- Use a nude-coloured eyeliner on your lower waterline if you have done a particularly smoky eye look to help open up the eye and make your eyes appear bigger.

- To make your eyeliner last longer on your waterline, apply the same colour in an eyeshadow on top. This will prolong its wear but make sure to dust off any excess powder to prevent irritating the eye.

- If you want a softer look then try using an eyeshadow instead of your liner as this will still give the eye a soft definition and is a great technique used with a smoky look.

- If you are a victim of your eyeliner transferring from your lash line to your eyelid crease, then try applying translucent powder to your eyelid or along the liner, depending on the intended finish. If you want a shiny black line then translucent powder will make it appear matte so instead keep your eye closed until the product has fully dried. Test it with a tap of a finger and once dry you can open your eye and do the other one.

- If you have small eyes, then refrain from lining the entire circumference of the eye as this will likely make the eye look smaller.

- If a precise line is too difficult then try drawing a rough line as close to the lashes as possible then use a cotton bud with makeup remover to sharpen up the edge before applying the rest of your eye makeup.

- Draw on your wing shape faintly first with an open eye but looking down into your mirror and then apply the rest of your liner from the inner corner to the outer, joining up to the wing shape. Follow the direction of your lower lash line and extend out towards your brow tail for the perfect shaped flick.

- Make your wing pop by applying some highlighter directly underneath the flick to make it stand out.

- More of a hack than a technique, try applying your pencil liner to the inside of your eyelash curler and when you curl your lashes the liner will print onto the eyelid for easy application. It's not the most precise technique and you may still have to draw over it but it is a great starting point and works really well.

- When creating a cat wing, try applying your liner from the outer corner of the eye and working inwards along the lash line to the middle then switch direction and pull the liner out from the inner corner.

- Try using a flick stamp for fail-safe wings. Simply adjust the angle of your stamp to suit your ideal shape.

Colour Choice

When it comes to eyeliner there is a vast array of colours. I have put together my favourite colours, that I think should be in everyone's makeup kit. However, if you only choose one colour for your kit then I would definitely recommend you go for a black. It is versatile, suits all eye shapes and it is always vivid and bold but can be softened with blending. Use a brown for a more subtle look and when creating soft smoky looks. Grey liner is good for brightening and softening the eye, but it is not a colour I have ever used on myself or a client. If you want to be super trendy then try using a navy, green or purple liner. White used to be popular in the 90s but is fantastic at making eyes look bigger when applied along the lower waterline; if you feel this is too bold, as it can sometimes look a bit over the top, then try using a nude instead for an instant eye-awakening effect that will hide any evidence of a heavy or late night. There are many glitter varieties too, for festive fantasy looks.

There is no right or wrong so have fun applying your graphic shapes, wings, flicks, ticks, dashes and dots with an endless choice of colour liners.

Recommended Brushes

Angled Brush

I personally use this brush shape for gel eyeliner as this gives me precision due to its short, angled shape and densely packed bristles. The angle is great for creating any eyeliner shape for both top and bottom lashes, waterlines and creating the eyeliner flick. I prefer this brush to an eyeliner brush as I often find the pointed shape of an eyeliner brush to be too flimsy and the bristles tend to be too long and therefore harder to control. If you want precision from your brush, I would always choose one with short, densely packed bristles.

Square Brush

Another brush I like to use is a square-ended brush for applying eyeliner. It is a small, thin rectangle-shaped brush with dense short bristles which gives good application control and can be used to stamp eyeliner along the lash line due to its equally square shape. I would not recommend doing graphic lines and flicks with this shape brush but for a tight line or a smudgy line, this brush is perfect.

EYE COLOURS

Forget the brushes, the brands, the types of product and even the techniques for now. The most important part of your makeup regime comes down to colour theory – the science behind which colours will suit you and why.

Colour theory is mentioned numerous times throughout this book in every aspect of the makeup regime from choosing your foundation shade, concealer, contouring, blusher, your lipstick and now your eye makeup.

Colour theory is so important, it is the ultimate key to unleashing your best eye makeup looks.

I am hopefully going to give you all the information you need so you can confidently choose the right colours to suit you, your eye colour and desired look.

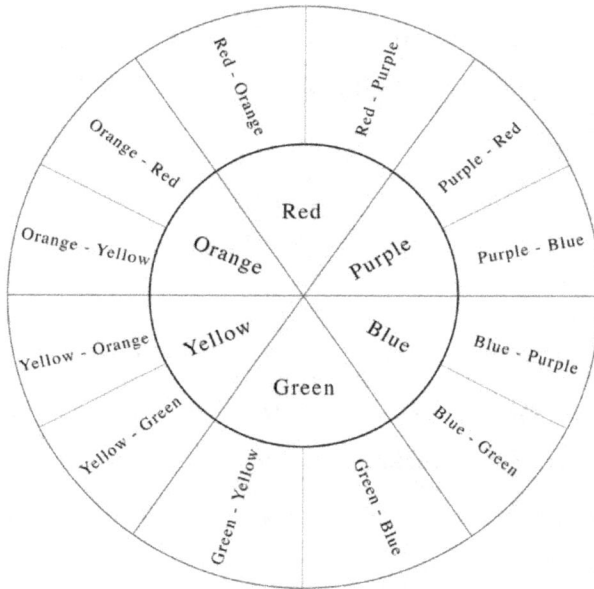

Colour theory normally forms quite a substantial part of a makeup course and is relevant to all aspects of the makeup regime from eyebrow to lips and is why I have mentioned it so much throughout my book.

When it comes to working with colour theory for eye makeup you want to remember that you are trying to enhance or complement your iris colour to make your eyes stand out and 'pop'.

I don't want to get you bogged down with too much colour theory jargon. As long as you understand your undertones, the basics of colour corrections, complementary/contrasting colours, i.e. opposite colours on the colour wheel and harmonising colours, then this is enough for you to make educated choices when it comes to choosing all your makeup products, colour correcting if needed and applying your ideal makeup look.

Complementary Colours

Complementary colours are the colours opposite one another on the colour wheel. For example, blue and orange are opposite each other on the wheel and therefore will complement each other. I work with complementary colours all the time when applying and designing makeup. A good example of this is colour correction; when carrying out colour corrections you use complementary colours as they will cancel one another out, e.g. if you have lots of blue tones in your skin, like dark circles under the eyes, then using an orange concealer is going to neutralize those tones, cancel them out and remove the dark circles. Another good example of how we use complementary colours in our everyday makeup is if you have a red spot or blemish, then applying a green concealer over the top will neutralise that redness.

When blue and orange are placed side by side, it creates a strong contrast. Complementary colours are also known as contrasting colours.

Harmonising Colours

Colours that lay next to one another on the colour wheel and that share one primary colour are known as harmonising colours. For example, blue, indigo and violet are next to each other on the colour wheel and they all share the common colour blue, therefore these are harmonising colours, which means that they blend easily into one another and that they work well side by side.

Choosing the Best Colour for You

When choosing your eye makeup, if you want your eyes to stand out then I recommend that you use complementary/contrasting colours – choose a colour that lies opposite your natural eye colour on the colour wheel.

Not only do you want to be working with your natural eye colour, you also can take your skin tone into consideration. If you have warmer tones in your skin then stick with warmer tones like peach, corals, reds and purples. If you have cool tones then stick with the tones like pink, blue and greens to help complement your makeup appearance further.

To work out the tone of your skin, read about understanding your skin tone, under the Foundation chapter.

Blue Eyes

People with blue eyes particularly suit the colour orange. Now, I don't want to scare anyone off by telling you that you must apply a bright orange eyeshadow – although it would look pretty cool, it wouldn't be to everyone's taste – instead think of the orange in a spectrum in terms of eyeshadows. So, think earth-toned shadows such as peach, warm browns, bronze, golds and copper eyeshadows. These tones will make blue eyes pop. You can wear blue eyeshadow on blue eyes but go for a deeper blue like navy or indigo which work really well to complement a blue eye.

Green Eyes

People with green eyes particularly suit purples and pinks. Again, you don't have to apply a Cadbury purple to your eyelid, unless you want to of course, but you could use a plum shade, mauve, lilac, light pink and rosy shades which will all really complement a green eye. Slate grey and black look beautiful on green eyes, as does silver and olive.

Brown Eyes

You're in luck! People with brown eyes tend to suit pretty much any colour but if you really want your eyes to stand out then try using a navy, dark blue, purple or gold eyeshadow.

Hazel Eyes

Hazel eyes tend to come in all shades, from golden brown to green brown, so you have got lots of options when it comes to choosing your eyeshadow. You can play up the different tones. Try enhancing the green tones by applying purple or pink shades of eyeshadow, or highlight the yellow tones by applying a metallic bronze. Experiment with some different tones and see what works for you.

You will be amazed at how your eyes can be transformed with just a simple swipe of colour.

In reality, there might be a colour you absolutely adore to wear, that might not be a complementary colour or perhaps doesn't suit your skin tone, but makeup is subjective. The most important thing is if you feel confident wearing it, then go for it. It is your makeup, colour theory is just a guide.

EYE MAKEUP BRUSHES

There are literally hundreds of different eye makeup brushes available on the market, which can make purchasing a brush a bit daunting, especially if you don't know what the brush shape actually does. Some brushes are named after their shape, some by their specific use and others are numbered. As a makeup artist, I do own a lot of brushes of all different sizes, shapes, types and colours and even I don't use them all! I want to share with you the main shapes of brushes that I like to use, what the different shapes actually do and which shape brushes you shouldn't be without for your own makeup kit.

I use a wide range of different brands of brushes in my professional and personal kit and purchase my brushes based on their shape to suit my needs. I often have duplicates of my favourite shapes and also have slight variations of certain shapes in my kit. I am not saying you need hundreds of brushes to be able to apply your makeup but there are particular shape brushes that I would highly recommend investing in to make your job quicker and easier when applying your eye makeup.

When it comes to choosing your brushes, it can be hard deciding what brushes you need and which brushes you will use. Often brushes are named after their shapes, i.e. angled brush, or they will be named after their function, i.e. concealer brush. Just because a brush is named after their main function does not mean it cannot be used elsewhere on the face so you may not need to have every single type of a brush as long as you have the essential shapes.

Angled/Brow Brush

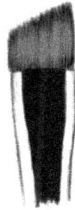

This is great for precision work and often used for brow defining and is suitable to be used with powder, pomades and gels. I personally use this brush shape for gel eyeliner as this gives me precision due to its short, angled shape and densely packed bristles.

Flat/Eyeshadow Brush

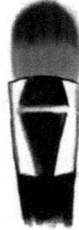

This is used for patting eyeshadow, cream and loose pigments onto the eyelid and general eye area. This brush shape comes in a variety of different sizes and thicknesses but fundamentally it does the same thing: apply eyeshadow. I use this type of brush all the time when applying any of my eyeshadows and really recommend you have this brush shape as an essential for your kit. This brush can be dampened to enhance the depth of colour shadow that you are applying.

Brow Brush/Comb

Also known as a spoolie, it looks like the end of a mascara wand. This is designed to comb through brows before applying brow products and can be used after to soften and blend the brows. I like to brush through my lashes with this brush before applying mascara and sometimes after to remove any clumps. This brush is great to use on false lashes too and helps separate the lashes on the strip before applying, and can then be used to combine the false lash to the real lashes for a seamless blend.

Crease Brush

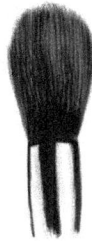

This brush shape is used to give a wash of colour to the eyelid, blending eyeshadows and for contouring and adding depth to eyes. I don't go anywhere without one.

I use the crease brush to blend my eyeshadow colours into the eye socket and to soften and blend the edges of my eye makeup on and around the eye. I also like to use this brush shape for buffing in cream concealer under the eyes to help soften them.

The crease brush comes in a variety of different sizes, the larger, rounder size of this brush is used for blending and applying washes of colours to a large area on the eye giving a softer, blended look.

This brush is also known as a blending brush and I love to use this shape for applying and blending eyeshadow washes into the crease of the eye.

The smaller size of brush is great for blending eyeliner, creating intense smoky eye looks and depositing more pigment of colour to a more precise area like the outer corner of the eyelid, or the lower lash line, for example.

There is another version of the crease brush which is angled instead of round but they do the same thing. I personally don't use the angled crease brush but this shape is good for beginners getting used to blending colours in the crease as this shape of brush naturally hugs the contours of the eye.

Pencil Crease Brush / Smudger Brush

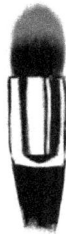

This is a smaller version of the crease brush which is slightly less fluffy than a crease brush and has shorter densely packed hairs. This brush is a good shape for depositing a depth of colour and blending the lower lash line and eyeliner and intensifying the outer corner of the eye. Use the larger crease brush to blend product further.

Fine Liner Brush

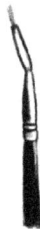

This brush shape is designed for applying liquid or gel eyeliner and is the perfect shape and size for creating the flick, however I rarely use this shape brush as I prefer to use the angled brush for applying my eyeliner.

Concealer Brushes

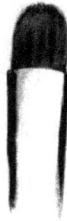

A concealer brush is used for applying cream and liquid concealer to the skin. The concealer brush looks similar to the flat eyeshadow brush but is usually slightly narrower. The dense shape makes it great for applying cream concealer and cream eyeshadows. The crease brush is also a great shaped brush for buffing and blending in your concealer into the skin.

As previously mentioned, you don't need to own millions of brushes to apply your makeup as a lot of brushes have multiple uses. Just make sure you clean them off between using them on different areas of the face or with different products so you don't end up muddying up your makeup.

For your eye makeup brush kit, I would suggest that you only need four brushes – an angled eyeliner brush, as it can be used for liner and brows, a flat eyeshadow brush, as this can be used for eye primer, eye base, eyeshadows and concealer, a round fluffy crease brush for blending and adding washes of colour to the eyes and blending your concealer and a smaller pencil crease brush for applying product on the lower or upper lash line and blending out eyeliner.

I do not like those sponge applicators that you get with eyeshadow palettes. They drag the skin, they are near impossible to clean properly and I do not recommend using them to apply your makeup, in fact just throw them away.

7. EYE SHAPES

IDENTIFY YOUR EYE SHAPE

There are many different eye shapes. It is worth identifying your eye shape to ensure that your makeup choice is working for your eye shape rather than against it.

Everyone has a unique eye shape, it is not a one size fits all, as sometimes an eye shape is made up from a combination of different shapes and settings.

The following is an overview of the different eye shapes, including their characteristics, to help you identify your eye shape. Once you have identified your eye shape then you can proceed to your individual eye shape chapter where you will find lots of techniques and tips to try and I will tell you what lash style and eyeliner shape is best suited for your eye shape.

Mono Lid

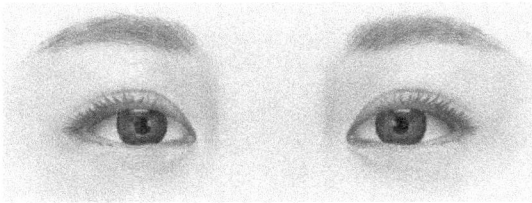

The mono lid eye has little to no natural crease. This is common in Asian eyes.

Turn to page 86.

Hooded Eye

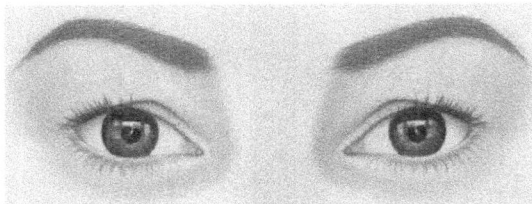

The hooded eye has very little visible eyelid and natural crease as it has an extra layer of skin that tends to fold to the lash line from the brow. This is common amongst mature people. Turn to page 93.

Upturned Eye

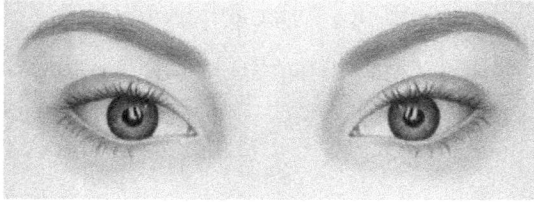

The upturned eye has a natural lift to the outer corners.

Turn to page 101.

Downturned Eye

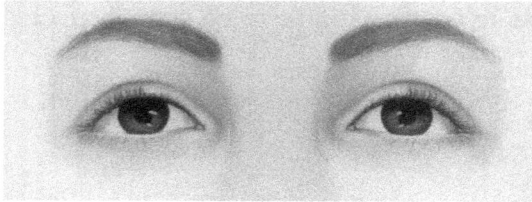

The downturned eye has a slight droop to the outer corners.

Turn to page 108.

Round Eye

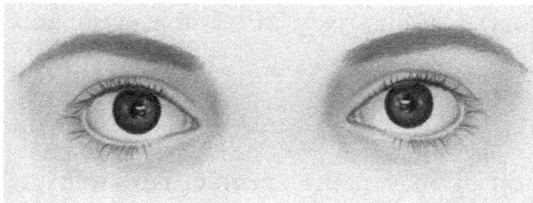

The round eye shape tends to be slightly larger and rounder than the almond eye. The whites of the eye are more visible around the iris, as is the natural crease of the eye.

Turn to page 115.

Almond Eye

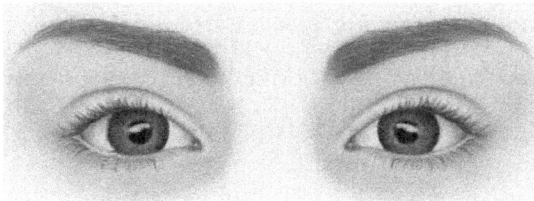

The almond eye resembles an almond in shape and is perfectly symmetrical with slightly upturned outer corners.

Turn to page 122.

Wide-set Eyes

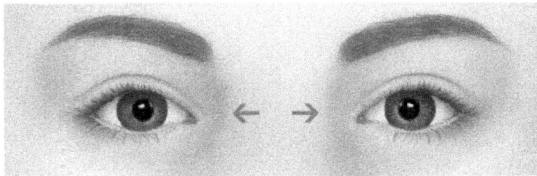

Wide-set eyes sits further apart on the face and can be identified by having more than one eyeball width in between the eyes.

Protruding Eyes

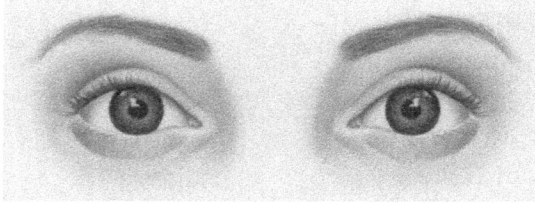

Protruding or bulging eyes are often quite large and they can bulge or protrude quite severely or only slightly. The eyes can be large or small.

Close-set Eyes

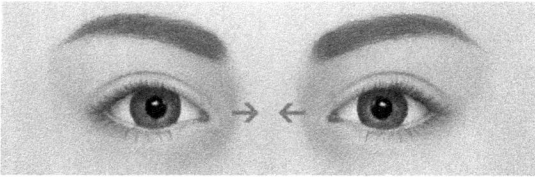

Close-set eyes sit closer together on the face with less than the width of your eyeball between them.

Deep-set Eyes

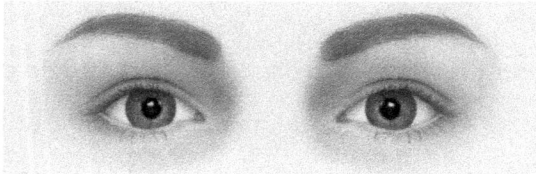

Deep-set eyes often sit deeper in the skull and accompany a prominent brow bone.

A good way to find out if your eye shape is upturned or downturned is to imagine drawing a straight horizontal line across your eye, straight across the pupil. If the outer edge of your eye is above the line then you have an upturned eye and if the outer edge drops below the line, then you have a downturned eye shape.

When deciding if your eyes are wide- or close-set, imagine trying to put another of your eye widths between your eyes. If you can't fit it between them then you likely have close-set eyes and if you can fit more than one width of your eye between your eyes then you likely have wide-set eyes.

MONO LID EYE SHAPE

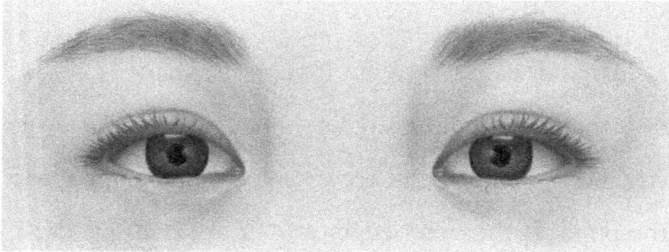

The mono lid eye has little to no natural crease, often a softer brow bone and is common in Asian eyes. Due to its spacious eyelid, it is suitable for multiple styles. When working with this eye shape, you want to concentrate on adding dimension, depth and definition.

Here is an overview of the mono lid eye shape including their characteristics, what lash and eyeliner style is best suited for your eye shape and some makeup techniques for you to try.

Look One (Day Look)

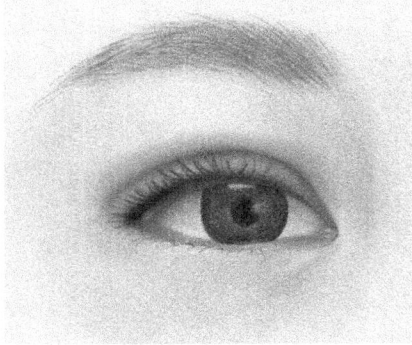

1) Prime and neutralise the eye area using an eye base or a skin-toned concealer and set with translucent powder or skin tone eyeshadow.

2) Apply a light shade across the entire eye area with an eyeshadow brush.

3) Using a medium shade and a crease brush, blend in a windscreen wiper motion above the eye lid to create the appearance of depth to create a false crease.

4) Line the upper lash line with a matte dark shade to define the eye. If there is a lot of visible lid then thicken the lash line but if there is not much visible lid, like a hooded

87

eye, then opt for a thinner liner that thickens out on the outer corners.

Look Two (Evening, Special Occasion)

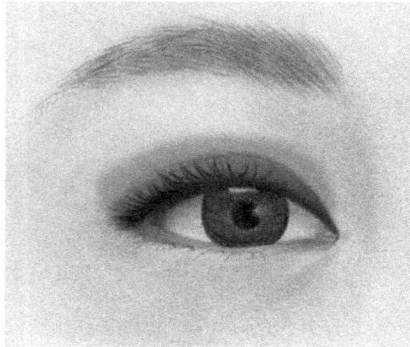

1) Prime and neutralise the eye area using an eye base or a skin-toned concealer and set with translucent powder or skin tone eyeshadow.

2) Apply a light matte eyeshadow shade all over the brow bone with a fluffy crease brush for a softer finish.

3) Apply a medium shimmery shade to the eyelid to maximise the lid space with a flat eyeshadow brush.

4) Apply a dark matte shade along the upper lash line with a pencil crease brush or square eyeliner brush and diffuse upwards to add definition.

Look Three (Every Day)

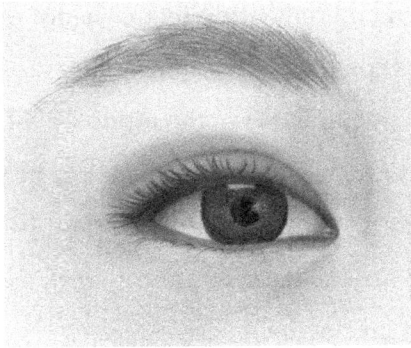

1) Prime and neutralise the eye area with an eye base or skin-toned concealer.
2) Apply a light shade across the brow bone with a fluffy crease brush for a softer finish.
3) Apply a medium matte shade to the entire lid with a flat eyeshadow brush.
4) Line the upper and lower lash lines with a dark matte shade using an angled eyeliner

brush and ensure the bottom lash line is thinner than the top.

When working with this eye shape you want to blend your shadows outwards and follow the natural flow of the lower lash line for the most flattering look.

I recommend only using matte shades on the brow bone and keeping the shimmery colours to the mobile lid to prevent emphasising the mono lid. Much like the hooded eye, we use matte shades to help minimise the appearance of the extra fold of skin. In this case, we want to use the darker shades to give the brow bone depth and create a false crease.

Using multi-layer lashes made up of a mixture of lengths, which is slightly on the heavier side, is best for this eye shape. The mixture of long and short hair in the false lashes will help create a wider, more open eye.

A dramatic cat eye or a graphic liner works really well with this eye shape. Make sure your eyeliner is thicker if there is a lot of lid space visible so it does not disappear when your eye are open. If the lid space is narrower then apply your eyeliner so that it gets thicker towards the outer corner. Smudge your liner upwards to create a slight smoky look or keep it really crisp, and ensure your eyeliner wings extend outwards at an upward angle.

A Smoky Eye for a Mono Lid Eye

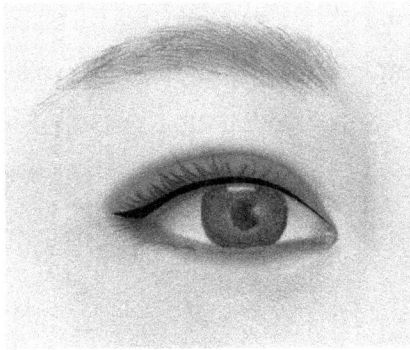

I love creating the traditional smoky eye with this eye shape, the dark intensity is across the lash line and blends up the eye instead of across the eye. You can use simple black eyeliner and a matte medium shade to create this look. You want to line the entire top lash line with your black liner and then blend your medium shade over the top of this whilst blending upwards to the brow bone, above the natural crease so it is visible when the eye is open. Mirror the same underneath the eye across the lower lash line.

Follow with your layered lashes and blend your eyeliner slightly upwards for a beautiful smoky style that will look great with your eye shape.

I recommend using a pencil crease brush for blending and intensifying the lash line and using a fluffy crease brush for blending to help soften and diffuse the colours. With smoky eyes, do not be afraid to use darker shades. When using darker shades I have always found it helps to apply lighter shades first, followed by the darker shades. In doing this, you can gradually build up the intensity and ensure that you do not end up with an overpowering result – remember, it is easier to add than it is to take away!

Don't forget to apply your mascara. I recommend doing your eye makeup first before applying your base, especially when doing a smoky eye, so that you can tidy up any fall out from the eyeshadows and you can easily neaten any edges with your base products.

Have fun trying out my techniques.

HOODED EYE SHAPE

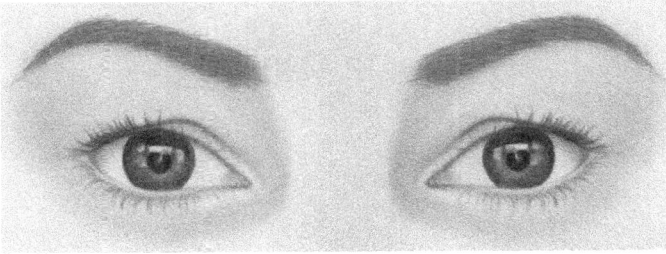

The hooded eye has very little visible eyelid and natural crease as it has an extra layer of skin that tends to fold to the lash line from the brow. When working with this shape you want to concentrate on enhancing the visible eyelid space.

The following is an overview of the hooded eye shape including their characteristics, what lash and eyeliner style is best suited for your eye shape and some makeup techniques for you to try.

Look One (Day Look)

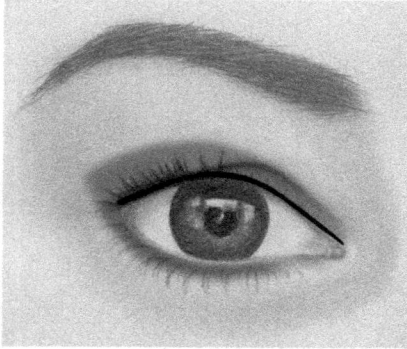

1) Prime and neutralise the eye area using an eye base or a skin-toned concealer and set with translucent powder or skin tone eyeshadow.

2) Apply a light shade of eyeshadow with a flat eyeshadow brush to the entire mobile lid to maximise the visible lid.

3) Blend a medium shade eyeshadow with a fluffy crease brush into the natural crease and buff and blend upwards using a windscreen wiper motion and ensure you blend up onto the brow bone.

4) Apply a darker matte shade to the top lash line and smudge and blend upwards.

Look Two (Evening, Special Occasion)

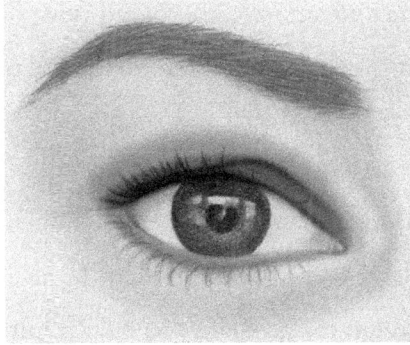

1) Prime and neutralise the eye area using an eye base or a skin-toned concealer and set with translucent powder or skin tone eyeshadow.

2) Apply a light shade of eyeshadow with a flat eyeshadow brush to the brow bone and inner corner of the eye and blend well.

3) Blend a medium shade eyeshadow across the entire mobile lid with a flat eyeshadow brush and using a fluffy crease brush to

blend into the natural crease, buff and blend upwards using a windscreen wiper motion and ensure you blend up onto the brow bone.

4) Apply a darker matte shade to the top lash line and smudge and blend upwards and outwards to the outer corner for more definition.

For a hooded eye you want to avoid using shimmery light colours on the brow bone and instead opt for medium matte shades to help minimise the appearance of the excess skin fold and give the eye some depth, which is what is lacking from a hooded eye. I have a hooded eye shape and for an everyday look I like to use a light to medium shade applied with a fluffy crease brush to my crease and brow bone and using the same brush, apply a medium to dark shade on the outer corner. I use a pencil crease brush to apply the same shade under the lower lash line. I then use a light shade, sometimes with a little shimmer, right to the centre of the eyelid and inner corner which helps open the eye. I find this gives my eyes lots of definition, the hood does not seem so severe and it is quick and easy to do before the school run.

When blending your eyeshadow, always blend upwards and allow the colour to be buffed above the natural crease so it is visible when the eye is open.

You must be very careful while choosing your false eyelashes for a hooded eye. With the wrong lash you run the risk of making your eyes seem small. I recommend using a fluttery style of lash with slightly longer fibres in the centre of the weft to help open up the eye.

A hooded eye means that there tends to be a small eyelid space to work with so you don't want to cover it all up with eyeliner. A thinner eyeliner that is tight to the upper lash line will work well and applying a flesh tone eyeliner to the waterline of the bottom lashes will help open out the eye further. A little trick I like to do to intensify my lash line is to apply eyeliner to the upper waterline, this helps lashes appear fuller and more voluminous without the liner taking over my makeup look.

Another good technique for eyeliner is to only apply your liner to the outer corner and blend it into the lashes a third of the way into the eye. If you want to apply eyeliner to the lower lash line then concentrate it on the outer corner and blend a third to prevent closing off the eye and making it appear small.

A Smoky Eye for a Hooded Eye

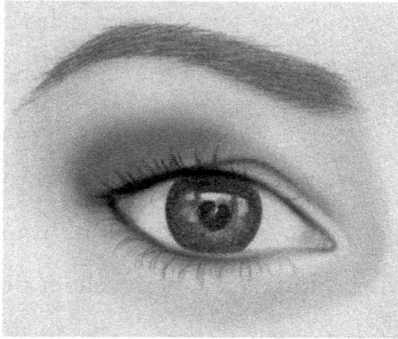

When creating a smoky look on a hooded eye, you want to refrain from applying a dark shade all the way across the eye as you could make the eye appear deeper set and smaller than it really is. I love creating the traditional smoky eye with this eye shape, the dark intensity is across the lash line and blends up the eye instead of across the eye. Use a matte taupe or medium shade on the natural crease and blend up the brow bone above the natural crease onto the hooded area so it is visible when the eye is open.

If you have a particularly small visible eyelid then I recommend, instead, using lighter highlighter colours on the centre of the lid and inner corner to help open up the eye. Blend the medium-dark shades three quarters of the way across the brow bone where the natural crease would be and taper off toward the inner corner of the eye using a windscreen wiper motion to diffuse and blend the tones together, creating the illusion of a crease and ensuring the makeup is visible.

Using the same shade, blend across the outer three quarters of the lower lash line with a pencil crease brush for added effect.

Follow with your fluffy lashes and choice of eyeliner for a beautiful smoky look that will look great with your eye shape.

I recommend using fluffy crease brushes for creating your smoky looks to help soften and diffuse the colours. With smoky eyes, do not be afraid to use darker shades. When using darker shades, I have always found it helps to apply lighter shades first, followed by the darker shades. This means you can gradually build up the intensity and ensure that you do not end up with an overpowering result – remember, it is easier to add than it is to take away!

Don't forget to apply your mascara. I recommend doing your eye makeup first before applying your base, especially when doing a smoky eye, so that you can tidy up any fall out from the eyeshadows and can easily neaten up any edges with your base products.

Have fun trying out my techniques.

UPTURNED EYE SHAPE

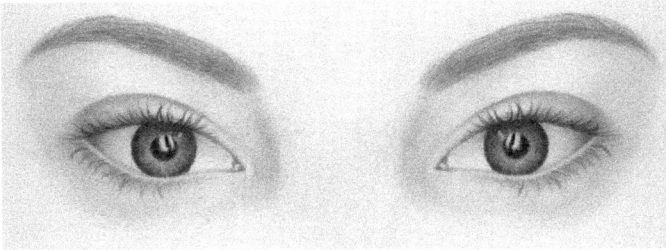

The upturned eye has a natural lift to the outer corners and is the perfect shape for creating smoky looks.

When working with this eye shape you want to concentrate on enhancing the lift and improving the symmetry.

Here is an overview of the upturned eye shape including their characteristics, what lash and eyeliner style is best suited for your eye shape and some makeup techniques for you to try.

Look One (Day Look)

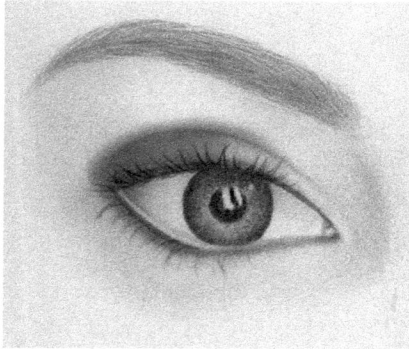

1) Prime and neutralise the eye area using an eye base or a skin-toned concealer and set with translucent powder or skin tone eyeshadow.

2) Divide the eye in half vertically, apply a light eyeshadow shade to the inner half and a medium shade to the outer half with a flat eyeshadow brush and use a fluffy blending brush to blend the two together so there is a transition between the colours.

3) Line the third upper and lower lash outer corners with a dark shade.

Look Two (Evening, Special Occasion)

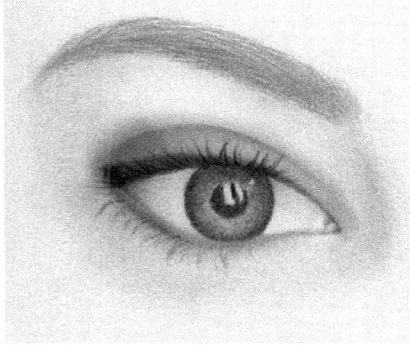

1) Prime and neutralise the eye area using an eye base or a skin-toned concealer and set with translucent powder or skin tone eyeshadow.

2) Apply a light shimmery eyeshadow shade all over the lid and inner corner with a flat eyeshadow brush or crease brush for a softer finish.

3) Apply a medium shimmery shade to the upper and lower lash lines with a pencil crease brush and blend upwards.

4) Apply a darker shimmery shade on the outer corner of the eye with a pencil crease

brush and blend outwards with a fluffy crease brush.

Look Three (Every Day)

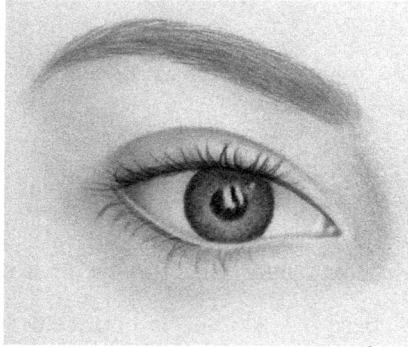

1) Prime and neutralise the eye area with an eye base or skin-toned concealer.

2) Apply a light shade across the brow bone with a fluffy crease brush.

3) Apply a shimmery light shade onto the mobile eyelid with a flat eyeshadow brush.

4) Line a third of the upper outer lash line with a dark thin line that is blended up.

5) Apply a thicker line to a third of the bottom outer lash line with the same shade and

blend out to enhance the symmetry of the eye.

Upturned eyes are already lifted so it is easy to emphasise and enhance this with eyeshadow and eyeliner. I recommend following the natural shape of the eye and playing up the upturned eye rather than trying to fight against it but it's entirely up to you.

The lower lid often appears longer than the top lid on an upturned eye so you can use your eyeliner or eyeshadow to balance out the eye shape by applying a straight thick line across the top lid and extending out straight on the outer corner of the eye. This will help minimise the natural lift. Apply a thick eyeliner to the bottom lashes from the middle of the iris to the outer edge of the eye and this will help keep the eye in proportion.

I recommend using flared half lashes applied to the outer corner to enhance this eye shape, however you can also use criss-cross lashes. The longer the style, the better for the most flattering look.

A Smoky Eye for an Upturned Eye

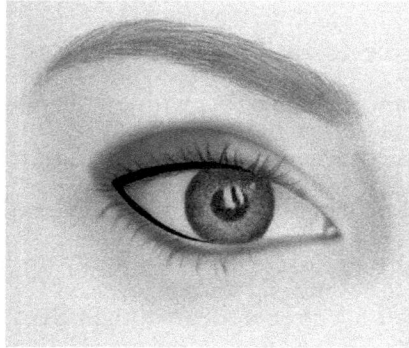

When creating a smoky eye look on an upturned eye, you want to split the eye in half and apply a lighter shade to the inner half of the eye and a darker shade to the outer half of the eye. Blend them well so there is transition between the tones, very much like Look One with the difference being the choice of shades. As we are going for a smoky look you can choose to use darker colours.

With the upturned eye, I like to emphasis the natural lift of the eye so I recommend following the natural flow of the lashes.

When creating a smoky eye, especially with an

upturned eye, I like to mirror what is on the eyelid across the lower lash line; the darker shade on the outer half and the lighter shade on the inner half. Make sure you blend the two together.

I recommend using fluffy crease brushes for creating your smoky look to help soften and diffuse the colours. With smoky eyes, do not be afraid to use darker shades. If using darker shades then I have always found it helps to apply lighter shades first, followed by the darker shades. In doing this, you can gradually build up the intensity and ensure that you do not end up with an overpowering result – remember, it is easier to add than it is to take away!

Don't forget to apply your mascara. I recommend doing your eye makeup first before applying your base, especially when doing a smoky eye, so that you can tidy up any fallout from the eyeshadows and can easily neaten up any edges with your base products.

Have fun trying out my techniques.

DOWNTURNED EYE SHAPE

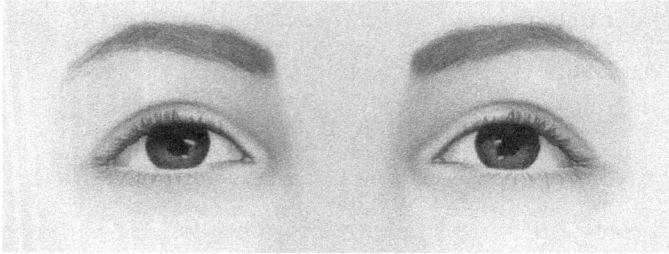

The outer corner of the eye turns downwards, hence the name a downturned eye. If you were to draw a straight line across your pupil, the outer corner would slightly drop below the line.

When working with this eye shape you want to concentrate on enhancing and lifting the outer corner of the eye.

Below, I have provided you with an overview of the downturned eye shape including their characteristics, what lash and eyeliner style is best suited for your eye shape and some makeup techniques for you to try, including a perfect smoky eye suitable for a downturned eye.

Look One (Day Look)

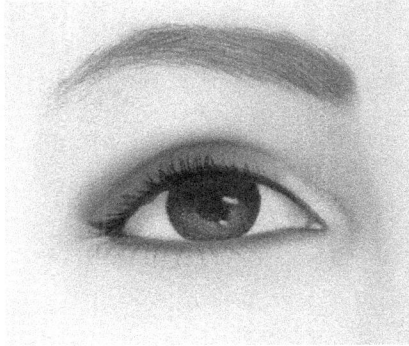

1) Prime and neutralise the eye area using an eye base or a skin-toned concealer and set with translucent powder or skin tone eyeshadow.

2) To lift the outer corner, apply a medium shade to the three-quarter outer corner, including the crease, and blend with a large crease brush.

3) Use a dark matte shade to line the outer corner of the upper lash line to help lift that downturn.

Look Two (Evening, Special Occasion)

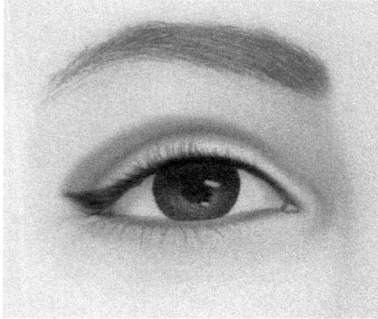

1) Prime and neutralise the eye area using an eye base or a skin-toned concealer, set with translucent powder or skin tone eyeshadow.

2) Apply a light shimmery shade across entire lid and blend up the brow bone with a rounded crease brush for a wash of colour.

3) Using the same brush, apply a medium shade to the natural eye crease and blend upwards towards brow.

4) To enhance the outer corner and help lift the shape, line the entire top lash line with your choice of eyeliner, from the inner corner right across to the outer corner. Start

to thicken the liner as you pass over the iris
and just before you get to the end of the
eye, where it starts to drop off, lift and
extend the liner in a slight wing to help lift
the eye further.

Look Three (Every Day)

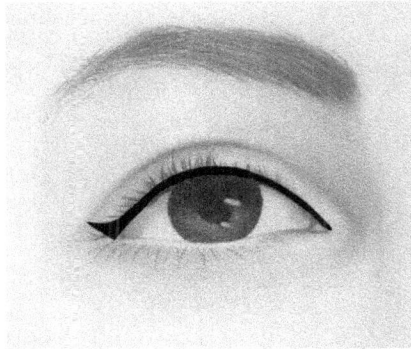

1) Prime and neutralise the eye area with an
   eye base or skin-toned concealer.
2) Apply a light shimmery shade across the
   mobile (the part that moves) eyelid using a
   flat eyeshadow brush.
3) Apply a matte light shade to the brow bone
   using a soft blending brush from crease to

brow.

4) Thinly line the entire upper lash line using an angled liner brush with a dark matte shade shadow or your choice of eyeliner, extending up and out on the outer corner. Do not apply liner to the bottom lash line.

These are all great looks to counteract your downturned eye. If you want to minimise the effect of the downturn then make sure that your eyeshadow and liner lift and extend on the outer corner or just before the eye starts to slant, and blend everything up and out to help counteract the downturn.

For downturned eyes, I recommend using flared false eyelashes to give you an attractive cat eye look. A flared lash will give your eyes a little lift and provide you with more balance.

The top lid often looks longer on this eye shape. The best eyeliner look to work with this eye shape is to apply a thin eyeliner from the inner corner of the top lash and thicken it as it moves towards the outer corner of the eye into a wing tip. This will help lift the edges of the eye upwards. I don't recommend applying eyeliner to the lower lash line, however adding a flesh tone liner to the waterline will help add further balance to the eye.

Smoky Eye for a Downturned Eye

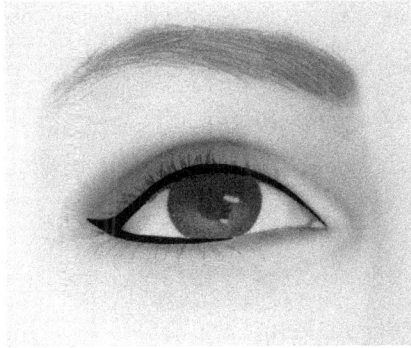

When creating a smoky eye look on a downturned eye, you want to minimise the downward slant by emphasising and lifting the corners of the eye. Try doing this by applying a bold cat eye shape. Make sure you extend the darker shade higher towards the brow bone along the outer three quarters of the upper lash line to help counteract that downward slant. Follow with your flared lashes and wing flicked eyeliner for a beautiful smoky style that will look great with your eye shape. I recommend using fluffy crease brushes for creating your smoky look to help soften and diffuse the colours.

With smoky eyes, do not be afraid to use darker shades. If using darker shades then I have always found it helps to apply lighter shades first, followed by the darker shades. In doing this, you can gradually build up the intensity and ensure that you do not end up with an overpowering result – remember our golden rule, it is easier to add than it is to take away!

Don't forget to apply your mascara. I recommend doing your eye makeup first before applying your base, especially when doing a smoky eye, so that you can tidy up any fall out from the eyeshadows and can easily neaten up any edges with your base products.

Have fun trying out my techniques.

ROUND EYE SHAPE

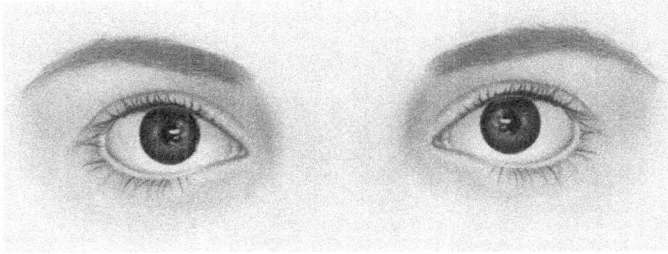

The round eye shape tends to be slightly larger and rounder than the almond eye. The whites of the eye are more visible around the iris, as is the natural crease of the eye. When working with this eye shape you want to concentrate on elongating the eye.

The following is an overview of the round eye shape including their characteristics, what lash and eyeliner style is best suited for your eye shape and some makeup techniques for you to try.

Look One (Day Look)

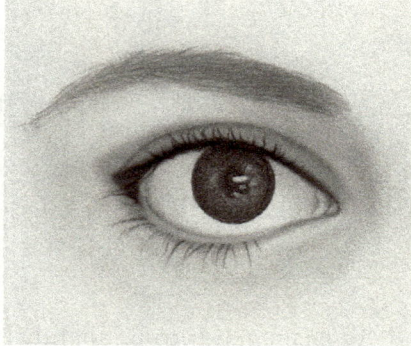

1) Prime and neutralise the eye area using an eye base or a skin-toned concealer and set with translucent powder or skin tone eyeshadow.

2) Apply a light shade to the mobile eyelid up to the natural crease using a flat eyeshadow brush.

3) Using a fluffy crease brush or pencil crease brush, apply a medium shade to the outer corner of the upper and lower lash line and blend in a circular motion. Sweep into a third of the crease to blend.

4) Use a dark matte shade to line the upper

lash line and blend at the corners to help extend and lift that outer corner to elongate the eye and counteract its roundness.

Look Two (Evening, Special Occasion)

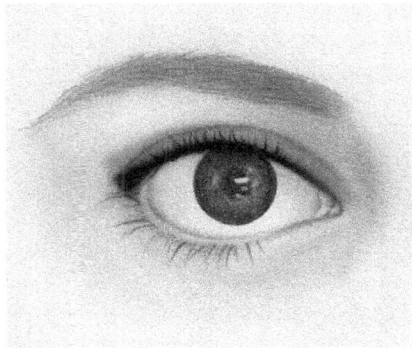

1) Prime and neutralise the eye area using an eye base or a skin-toned concealer, set with translucent powder or skin tone eyeshadow.
2) Apply a dark shade to the upper lash line and blend with a pencil crease brush to diffuse the colour.
3) Sweep a medium shade into the crease using a large fluffy crease brush and blend.
4) Apply a black eyeliner or shadow across the

entire upper lash line to accentuate your
round eyes.

Look Three (Every Day)

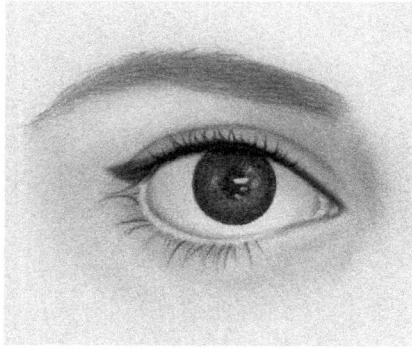

1) Prime and neutralise the eye area with an
   eye base or skin-toned concealer.

2) Apply a light shimmery shade across the
   mobile (the part that moves) eyelid using a
   flat eyeshadow brush.

3) Apply a matte medium shade to the eyelid
   with a flat eyeshadow brush.

4) Using a fluffy crease brush, sweep a matte
   pale shade across the entire brow bone and
   blend.

5) Line the outer corner of the eye with a dark shade using an eyeliner brush to emphasis the outer corner.

If you are trying to counteract or de-emphasise a round eye, you want to focus the most intensity on the upper lash line and use lighter shades on the lower lash line. Concentrate on blending your shadow up and out at the edges of the eyes to help lift and elongate the shape of the eye. For more drama, use a dark shade on the outer third of the lower lash line and blend up into the upper lash line for a beautiful smoky look.

Most of the false eyelash types and shapes will suit a round eye, however a criss-cross style of lash would look the best.

A longer winged eyeliner look will suit this eye shape by adding width and bringing attention to the outer corner. Start your liner a third of the way from the outer corner, starting off thin and thicken as the lash line meets the iris and extend out into a horizontal flick.

A Smoky Eye for a Round Eye

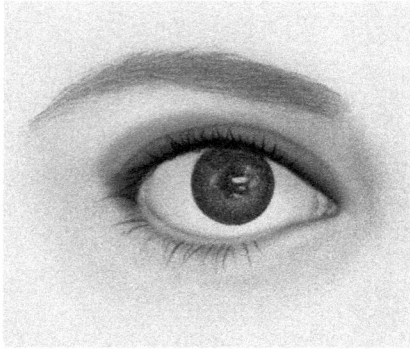

The goal when working with a round eye is to elongate the eye to counteract or de-emphasise its roundness. Your ideal smoky eye look is pretty much the same as Look Two for evening wear. Apply a light shade to the inner corner of the eye and blend to the mid lid. Next, use a medium shade on your lids, middle and outer corner and blend upwards into the crease. Apply the darkest shade along your upper lash line, working from the outside in and blend this colour up into the crease too. Apply the same dark shade across your lower lashes. If you have larger round eyes then you will be able to get away with applying the dark shade across the entire lash line which will make your eyes appear smaller but without closing them off. Stick to applying the dark shade to the outer third if you have a smaller round eye shape and blend that dark shade up and out into the upper lash line for a beautiful smoky look.

Don't forget to apply your mascara. I recommend doing your eye makeup first before applying your base so that you can tidy up any fall out from the eyeshadows and can easily neaten up any edges with your base products.

Have fun trying out my techniques.

ALMOND EYE SHAPE

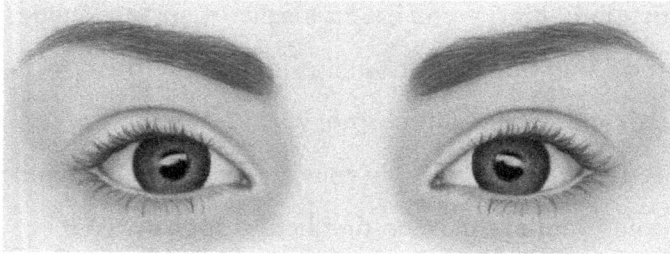

The almond eye resembles an almond in shape and is perfectly symmetrical with slightly upturned outer corners.

This eye shape is considered to be the most versatile and can carry off any look, however when working with this eye shape you want to concentrate on adding depth and intensity.

The following is an overview of the almond eye shape, including its characteristics, what lash and eyeliner style is best suited for your eye shape and some makeup techniques for you to try to get the most out of your almond eye.

Look One (Day Look)

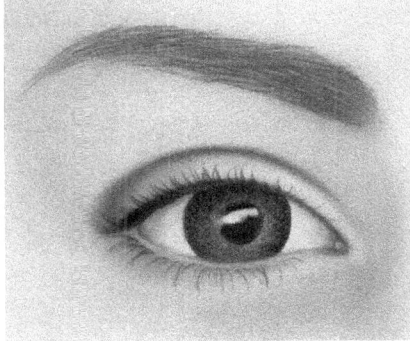

1) Prime and neutralise the eye area using an eye base or a skin-toned concealer and set with translucent powder or skin tone eyeshadow.

2) Apply a light matte shade to entire lid and blend just past natural crease using a flat eyeshadow brush.

3) Add depth by applying a medium shade to the outer three quarters corners using a crease brush and blend.

4) Using a pencil crease brush blend a darker matte shade across the top and bottom lash lines. If you have small eyes then I suggest

that you only line the outer three quarters
of the lower lash line to prevent closing off
your eye and making it seem smaller.

Look Two (Evening, Special Occasion)

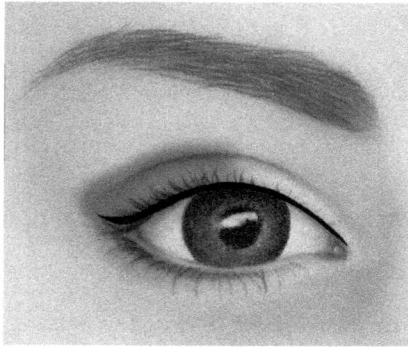

1) Prime and neutralise the eye area using an
   eye base or a skin toned concealer, set with
   translucent powder or skin tone eyeshadow.
2) Apply a light shade across entire lid and
   brow bone with a rounded crease brush for
   a wash of colour.
3) Using the same brush apply a medium
   shade to the natural eye crease in a
   windshield wiper motion to add depth and

blend it across the top lash line to create a V-shape.

4) Accentuate the outer corner by applying a darker shade to the outer crease with a pencil crease brush and blend in small circles to pull the colour out and upwards towards the temple for instant eye lifting effect.

Look Three (Every Day)

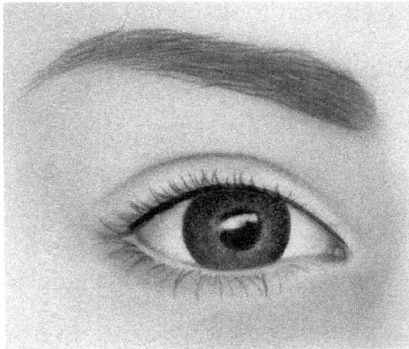

1) Prime and neutralise the eye area with an eye base or skin toned concealer.

2) Apply a light shimmery shade across the

mobile (the part that moves) eyelid using a flat eyeshadow brush.

3) Apply a matte light shade to the brow bone using a soft blending brush from crease to brow.

4) Using a pencil crease brush apply a medium to dark matte shade along the top lash line to give the appearance of a larger eye and apply liner to the upper waterline for instant lash thickening effects.

These are all great looks to enhance your almond eyes, you want to be emphasising and accentuating that natural uplift with this eye shape. Lift 'wing out' your eyeshadow at the outer corners along with your liner and blend everything up and away from the eye towards the temple for a visually lifting effect.

These are guidelines and you can interpret them how you wish. If you want to use shimmery shades then why not, if you want to rock an evening look during the day then go for it.

Anything goes when it comes to eyeliner for an almond eye but I recommend you pay attention to how much of the eyelid is visible as this will determine how thick your eyeliner should be. If you can see lots of lid then a thicker eyeliner will work just fine and don't be afraid to play up that natural uplift of your eye shape with a raised wing. If you don't have much of an eyelid, due to a prominent brow for example, then you may want to stick with a thinner lined eye but still extend those corners for some drama.

When it comes to choosing your lashes to suit your eye shape, you are in luck as an almond eye suits all shapes of lashes. You can simply choose the lashes that will suit your desired look whether that be natural and fluffy or something more va va voom and glam.

A Smoky Eye for an Almond Eye

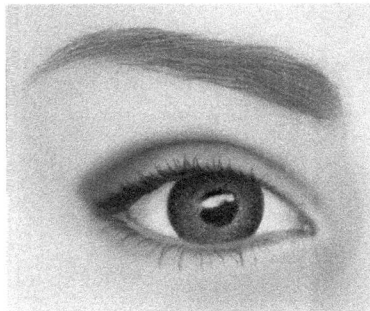

Apply a light shade across the entire lid from lash line to brow, use a medium shade on the outer edge of the eye in a V-shape and blend into the natural crease inwards towards the inner corner. Use a darker shade right on the outer edge of the lash line and blend outwards towards the temples to accentuate the eye shape.

Don't forget to apply your mascara. As always, I recommend doing eye makeup first before applying your base so that you can tidy up any fallout from the eyeshadows and can easily neaten any edges with your base products.

Have fun creating your almond eye looks.

EYE SETTINGS

When designing your eye makeup, it is important to understand your eye shape and their natural setting (where the eyes sit on the face) to ensure that your makeup is working for your eye shape rather than against it.

It is important to remember that when looking at

an eye shape, we are not only looking at the overall shape of the eye but where they are situated on the face too.

In this chapter you will find all my hints, tips and tricks to help you identify your eye setting and be able to make the most suitable choices when it comes to choosing your perfect style of eye makeup, including a smoky eye.

Everyone has a unique eye shape so it is not a one size fits all as the eye shape is made up from a combination of different shapes and settings. Below is an overview of the different eye settings, including their characteristics, to help you identify your eye setting, what lash and eyeliner style is best suited for your eye setting and the perfect smoky eye for your eye setting. If you would like to find out more about your eye shape, then please refer to the chapter containing your individual eye shape.

Deep-set Eyes

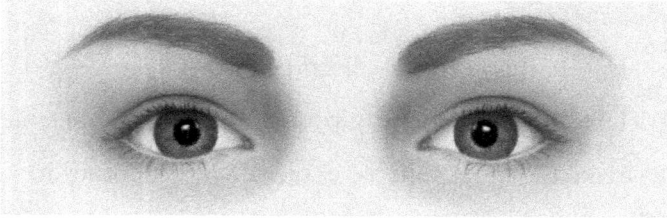

The deep-set eye often sits deeper in the skull and accompanies a prominent brow bone. When working with this eye shape, you want to enhance the eyelid and bring the eyes forward on the face.

For a deep-set eye, I recommend using long and wispy lashes as this shape of lash will create the appearance of an eye that is shallower. If you want to make your eyes look bigger then use lashes that get longer in the centre of the weft.

This eye setting can make the eyes appear smaller so you want to avoid using thick eyeliner. Instead, use a thin line across the top lashes and concentrated on the outer corner with a horizontal flick, if that's your thing. I recommend only applying your liner to three quarters of the lash line and blending it out to be more concentrated on the outer corner for a more sultry look. You do not need to apply any eyeliner into the inner corner of the eye, this would risk closing off the eye and making it seem smaller. You can have large eyes that are deep-set as well as small so you want to make sure that you are not working against your natural eye shape.

If you have larger deep-set eyes then you can add more width to your eyeliner on the outer edge so you can get away with a bigger wing.

A Smoky Eye for a Deep-set Eye

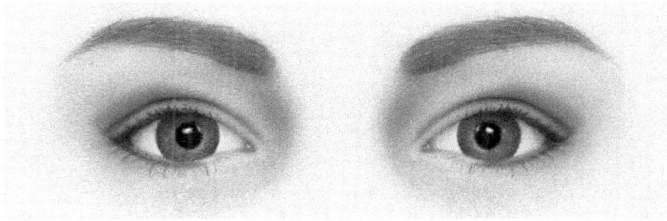

The goal when creating a smoky look on a deep-set eye is to bring the eyes forward whilst pushing the brow bone back. This can be achieved by using matte medium shades across the natural crease blended up the brow bone to help minimise the prominent brow. Apply your lightest shade to the mobile eyelid and inner corner to help bring the eyes forward whilst making your eyes appear larger. Blend the medium shade under the lower lash line ensuring you taper off towards the inner corner to prevent closing down the eye and making it seem smaller than it is.

Follow with long wispy lashes and apply your eyeliner across three quarters of the upper and lower lash lines for a beautiful smoky look that will look great with your eye setting.

Close-set Eyes

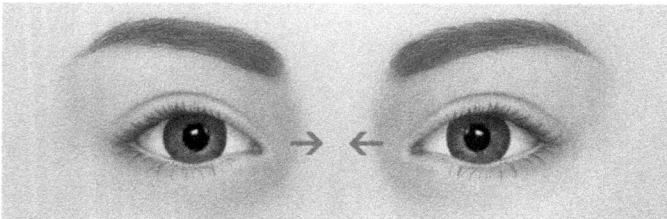

The close-set eye sits closer together on the face. When working with this eye shape, you want to concentrate on enhancing the outer corners to make the eyes appear further apart. A gradient eye makeup is best, something that transitions from light to dark across the eye. The lightest colour should be on the inner corner and mid lid, and the darker tones concentrated on the outer corner and blended into the crease. Add an extra pop of highlight into the inner corner and apply your mascara, sweeping the lashes out on the outer edges.

A long and voluminous criss-cross style of lash works well for this kind of eye setting. The criss-cross lashes will create the appearance of bigger eyes and will perfectly frame your eyes.

Apply your liner thinly towards the inner corner of the eye and thicken it as you get to the outer corner. Focus your eyeliner with the shadow on the outer part of the eye to pull the eyes further apart on the face.

A Smoky Eye for Close-set Eyes

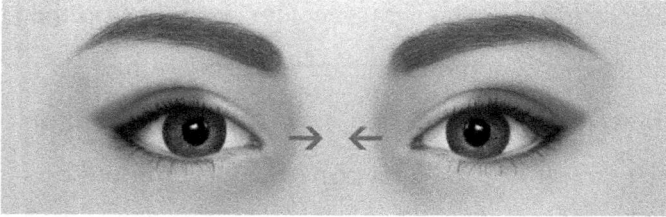

The goal when creating a smoky look on a close-set eye is to create the appearance that your eyes are further apart than they naturally are. This is best achieved by applying a gradient, something that transitions from light to dark across the eye. The lightest colour needs to be on the inner corner and mid lid, and the darker tones concentrated on the outer corner and blended across into the crease and along the lash line. Blend the darker shade up and out on the outer corner to elongate the eye and bring focus to the outer corner.

Follow with long wispy lashes and apply your eyeliner across three quarters of the upper and lower lash lines for a beautiful smoky look that will look great with your eye setting.

Wide-set Eyes

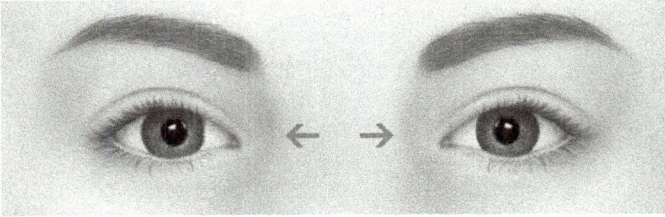

When it comes to determining if you have a wide-set eye, ask yourself this question: can you get more than one of your eyeballs between your eyes? If the answer is yes, then you likely have wide-set eyes. You want to create the appearance that your eyes are closer together. This can be achieved by using darker shades of eyeshadow across the eye, which can be applied to the inner corner too, unlike the close-set eye where we concentrate the darkness on just the outer corner. With this eye shape you want to apply it to the interior of the eye as well. A halo eyeshadow would work well to give the illusion of closer set eyes.

Apply your liner from the inner corner and extend across the entire lid. You could create a reverse cat eye and really define the inner corner of the eye with your liner.

When it comes to lashes, you want to go with a longer, fuller lash as this will help fill the space between your eyes, giving the appearance of closer set eyes.

A Smoky Eye for Wide-set Eyes

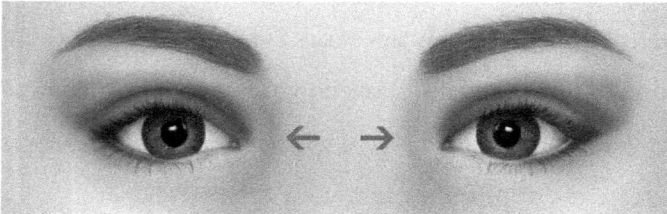

The goal when creating a smoky look on wide-set eyes is to create the appearance that your eyes are closer together than they naturally are. This is best achieved by applying medium shades to the inner half of the eye and using lighter shades on the mid lid and outer edges. You need to make sure everything is blended inwards towards the inner corner of the eye. As mentioned before, a halo eye makeup is a perfect smoky technique to use for this eye setting. The halo eye technique is when the crease, inner and outer corner are the same dark shade and a lighter shimmery shade is applied to the centre of the lid so it is surrounded on all sides by a darker shade. This is then mirrored on the lower lash line.

Follow with long, full lashes and apply your eyeliner across the entire upper lash line for a beautiful smoky look that will look great with your eye setting.

Prominent Eyes

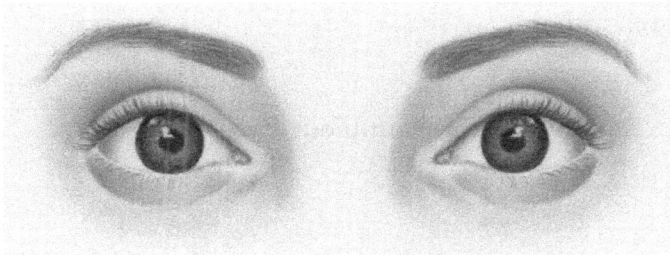

Prominent, also known as a protruding or bulging, eyes are often quite large, can bulge or protrude quite severely or only slightly and can give the appearance of a baby doll look. When working with this eye shape you want to concentrate on minimising the effect of the protrusion and the larger eye shape. This can be achieved by using matte darker tones of eyeshadow and I recommend lining the entire eye, either with a graphic or smudged liner to further give the appearance of a shallower eye. If you want to add lift to the eye then flick the outer corner of your liner upwards towards the tail of your brow.

If you want to play up a large eye, do the opposite by minimising the liner and using light, neutral colours or shimmery shades instead to add emphasis. Cluster lashes or a spikey style of strip lash with thicker and thinner lashes across the band will work well with this eye shape.

A Smoky Eye for Prominent Eyes

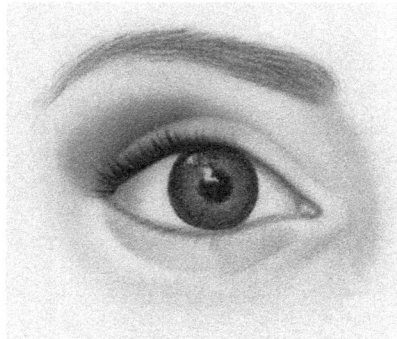

When working with a prominent eye, you want to create the effect of pushing the eye back and bringing the brow forward this can be achieved by applying a medium to dark matte shade to the middle of the eyelid and blending out across the eye, into the crease. A lighter shade can be applied to the inner corner to open up the eye and across the brow bone to bring this forward. Mirror the same technique across the lower lash line.

Follow with your spikey cluster lashes and apply your eyeliner thickly across the eyelid and blend outwards for added lift for a beautiful smoky appearance that will look great with your eye setting.

I recommend using a pencil crease brush for blending and intensifying the lash line, and using fluffy crease brushes for blending to help soften and diffuse the colours. With smoky eyes, do not be afraid to use darker shades. If using darker shades then I have always found it helps to apply lighter shades first, followed by the darker shades. In doing this, you can gradually build up the intensity and ensure that you do not end up with an overpowering result – remember the golden rule, it is easier to add than it is to take away!

Don't forget to apply your mascara. I recommend doing your eye makeup first before applying your base, especially when doing a smoky eye, so that you can tidy up any fall out from the eyeshadows and can easily neaten any edges with your base products.

Have fun trying out my techniques.

8. SMOKY EYES

The question I ask my clients most is: what type of smoky eye would you like?

There are lots of different techniques that can be used to create a smoky eye. You can create a simple smoky using just one colour of eyeshadow or eyeliner, you can create a gradient look that has the smokiness/darkness along the lash line for a true smoky eye or at the outer corner for a more modern look.

In this section of the book, I am going to give you lots of techniques, hints and tips that you can use to create a variety of smoky eye looks. If you want to find a smoky look that will suit your eye shape then please read the previous chapter on your eye shape where you will find your ideal smoky eye with techniques on how to create different looks that will suit your eye shape.

A smoky eye has to be one of my all-time favourite looks to create because they are so versatile, unique and sexy. They can be suitable for all occasions from the everyday or evening and can be glammed up for nights out and special occasions. I think I could write an entire book on its own about the variations of a smoky eye.

There are so many elaborate tutorials and eyeshadow products out there for creating smoky looks that it can seem somewhat daunting to even begin to contemplate creating a smoky eye. You may think it takes a long time and requires lots of products, colours and brushes but I am here to show you that this is not the case. You can easily create beautiful yet simple smoky looks using just one, two or three colour eyeshadows to create a variety of different smoky looks.

One Colour Smoky

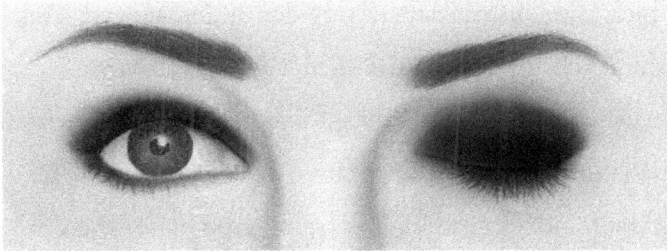

This has to be one of the simplest yet effective looks to create using just one product: your trusty black eyeliner.

This is one product I would never be without especially when creating any smoky look.

It is exactly what it says on the tin, it is one colour all over the eyelid. This can be applied in a variety of different shapes. You can blend the edges up and out to create a winged look or blend up past the natural crease onto the brow bone or keep purely on the mobile lid, it is up to you and depends on your desired look.

As always, make sure you are doing your eye makeup first before applying base products to your skin for easy clean up afterwards.

A simple trick to help with that dreaded fallout (when eyeshadow drops under the eye) is to apply a thick layer of translucent powder under the eye. This will catch the fallout and then this can easily be brushed off with little mess. You can also use eye pads or the cheaper alternative of cotton pads, folded in half and secured with masking tape under the eye to catch any fallout that may happen when using those darker colours.

Apply your concealer to the entire eye area to neutralise any discolouration, veins, dark circles, etc. Then set with a translucent powder or skin-toned eyeshadow powder to prevent the concealer or eye base from creasing.

Sharpen your pencil eyeliner and roll it into the palm of your hand to warm up the formula for easier application. Draw a line as close as you can to the entire lash line, this does not need to be neat as you will be blending it in anyway. Draw along the top and bottom lash lines, if you have small eyes then don't line across the entire length of the eye and just concentrate on the outer third to prevent closing off your eye and making them appear smaller.

Using a pencil crease brush, or smudger as they are often called, blend across the eyeliner in a windscreen wiper motion keeping in contact with the skin. Sweep back and forth over the top of that liner to blend it out, this may be enough smoke for you but if you want the entire eyelid to be smoky then you can colour in the entire eyelid with your eyeliner. Make sure you stop before the natural crease of the eye to leave enough space to blend otherwise you may run the risk of overdoing the blending and end up looking like a raccoon.

Another thing to try is once you have blended that liner across your lash line and you want more smoke, apply a black eyeshadow over the top, patting the colour onto the mobile lid with an eyeshadow brush or shader brush, as it's sometimes known as, but stay clear of the natural crease at this point. Switch to a fluffy crease brush and blend that shadow up the mobile lid and into the crease and outwards to elongate the eye, if needed.

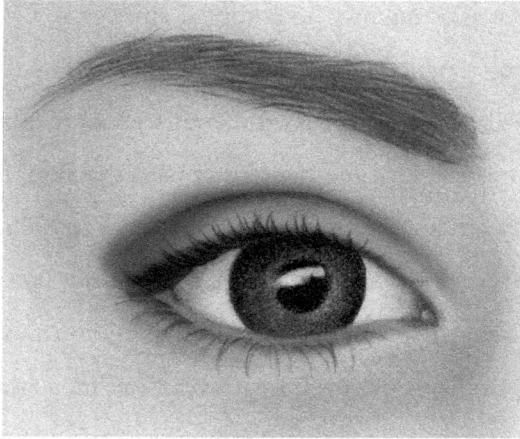

Another technique or look you can create using just one colour is to apply your choice of colour shadow to the outer corner of the eye in a sideways V-shape with a fluffy crease brush or pencil crease, and blend this colour into the natural crease using a windscreen wiper motion to blend. Apply the same colour along the upper lash line and sweep it along the lower lash line, then apply your favourite mascara and you are good to go. It's an easy smoky eye to create.

Don't forget to apply lashings of your favourite mascara or apply a set of voluminous lashes. Apply your pencil eyeliner along your waterlines on the top and bottom to give you some added smoke.

Why not try using aubergine, navy or olive green for creating a smoky eye instead of using black or brown for a beautiful sultry look.

True Smoky (Gradient – Up the Eye)

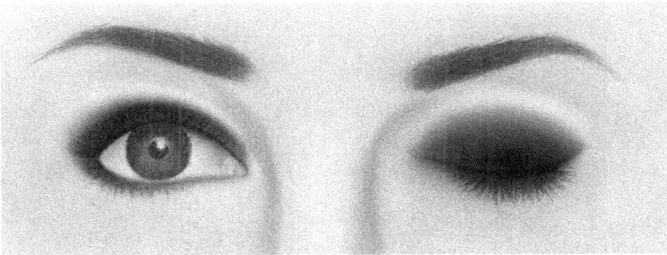

A true smoky eye is when the intensity of the colour or darkness is across the lash line and blends up the eye towards the crease much like the one colour, although with this technique you apply the black eyeliner and shadow onto the entire lid. With the true smoky eye, you apply the colour right along the lash line and blend it up so it softens whilst going up the eye.

Neutralise the eye with concealer, set with a translucent powder or skin-toned eyeshadow.

Using a pencil eyeliner or shadow draw across the entire lash line, top and bottom and blend using a pencil crease brush. If you find too much product is travelling and making a mess, try swapping to a clean crease brush or a bigger fluffier crease brush and blend with that instead. Another trick to try is to dip your brush in translucent powder and buff this over the top of your eyeliner or shadow to help blend the colours without depositing any further product across the eyelid.

Two Colour Smoky

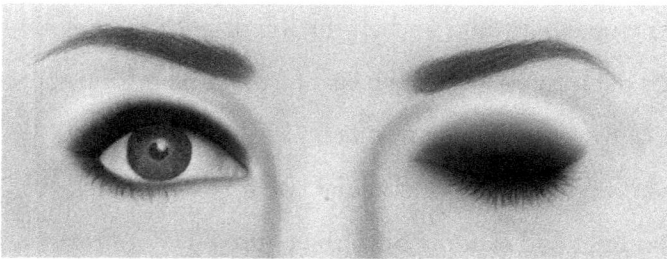

For this two colour version of a smoky eye you are only using a dark shade and a medium transition, blending shade. Apply the medium shade with a fluffy crease brush in a windscreen wiper motion to the natural crease of the eye, on the outer corner of the upper eye and along the lower lash line.

Apply your dark shade onto the mobile lid with a flat eyeshadow brush, then use the same crease brush to blend this dark colour into the medium shade you have already applied to diffuse and soften those edges. You can also apply the dark shade first, just make sure you blend it out before applying the medium shade to prevent muddying the colours or blending it too far. Use a flat eyeshadow brush to apply the dark shade onto the mobile lid, blend with a fluffy brush and use the same brush to pick up the lighter colour and buff and blend this onto the outer edges of the dark shade and blend into the crease to create an ombre effect.

Apply black eyeliner to the top and bottom waterlines for added drama.

Gradient (Across the Eye)

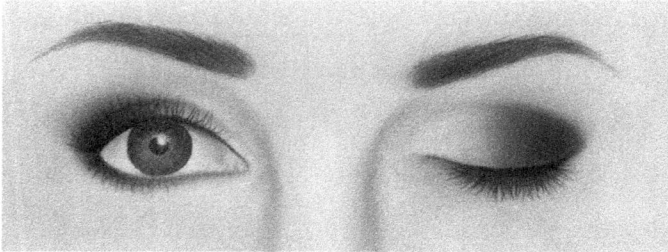

This is probably the most common technique that I use when creating my eye looks and is not only reserved for creating smoky eye. I use this technique 90% of the time with my clients and I think is the most versatile and flattering of the looks as it can be tailored to suit all eye shapes with a little tweaking.

The gradient eye is when the eyeshadow colour transitions from light to dark across the eye and is predominantly darker on the outer third of the eye and blended into the natural crease. It's a perfect style for deep-set and downturned eye shapes. This technique can easily be adapted to suit an upturned eye by dividing the eye in half and applying the darker shade to the outer half. This is the most involved technique which requires lots of blending so start off softly with the lighter colours and build up to the darker colours. This will likely require lots of practice so here is a step-by-step guide to make it easier:

1) Neutralise the eye area with a skin-toned concealer, set with translucent powder or skin-toned eyeshadow to stop the concealer or eye base from creasing.

2) Choose your choice of colours (refer to the Eye Colours Section for information on colours that will help make your natural eye colour stand out).

3) Apply the lightest colour to the inner corner and inner quarter of the eyelid using an eyeshadow brush to pat on the colour.

4) Apply your transition shade (darker than your lightest colour but lighter than your darkest colour) with a fluffy crease brush to the outer third of the eye in a V-shape and blend into the upper lash line, into the natural crease and slightly onto the brow bone if you have a hooded eye.

5) Apply the same shade three quarters along

your lower lash line and blend up and out into the upper outer lash line.

6) Apply your darkest shade using a smaller pencil crease brush and, using small circular movements, apply on top of the V shape you created with the transition shade and blend. Use the larger fluffy crease brush and blend this shade across the upper lash line, the outer corner and inwards towards the nose in the natural crease. Dip your brush in translucent powder before you do any blending to help prevent the colours from travelling too far.

7) Apply the same dark shade to the outer edge of the lower lash line with a small pencil crease brush and blend in towards the inner corner. You want to mirror what is on the upper lid to the bottom lid, but you can make it more smoky and intense by applying the dark shade all the way across the lower lash line or perhaps picking a different colour all together, it is up to you and depends on your desired look.

8) Apply your choice or eyeliner shape to the

upper lash line and lower lash line.

9) I recommend applying eyeliner to the upper water line and lower water line if you are using darker colours. If you have used this technique but are using softer lighter colours then you may not need to apply your liner to the lower waterline, instead opt to use a skin tone liner to really help open that eye out.

10) Apply your favourite mascara on the top and bottom lashes and apply some lashes if you like.

You can adapt this look with any colour combinations, you just need to make sure you have three colours: light, medium to use as your transition blending shade and a darker shade for definition and intensity. You can add foil, cream shadows, glitter and even use bright colours.

This technique is the most universal and with small tweaks can be made to suit any eye shape and suit any occasion, it just takes practice and your inspiration, so give it a go.

Recommended Brushes and Tools

Please refer to the chapter on eye makeup brushes to see my recommended brushes that I like to use when creating beautiful smoky eyes.

Tips on Applying Your Smoky Eyes

- Don't forget to do your eye makeup first before applying any base products for an easier clean and tidy up. Use cotton buds and makeup remover to clean up any wobbly edges.

- Neutralise and set your eyes to give yourself a blank canvas to work on to make your products last longer and have better vibrancy.

- Creating a smoky eye is all about blending, use a transition shade or nude eyeshadow to help with blending those darker colours.

- Don't use a waterproof eyeliner on your waterline as it will not draw and will require multiple applications which may cause unwanted irritation.

- Use flat brushes to pat on colours and use soft fluffy brushes for blending. The smaller the brush, the more intense the colour payoff will be.

- Apply translucent powder under your lower lash line to prevent your eyeliner or shadow from slipping.

- Spray your eyes with a setting spray before applying your mascara to prevent smudging.

- Less is more when it comes to creating smoky eyes and blending is key. You can always add more product if and when it is needed to prevent overdoing it.

- Apply a brown shade over the top, even if you are using black, for a more multi-dimensional diffused look.

- Keep the smoky colours next to the lashes and don't extend too far down past the lower lashes otherwise it can end up looking ghoulish.

- Try to avoid applying the dark shades right into that inner corner in the tear duct, instead opt for a highlighting light shade to help open the eye up and give your makeup that professional finish.

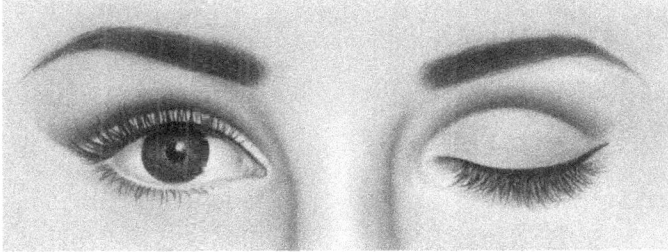

9. THE CUT-CREASE

Cut-crease is a makeup technique used to define the eye crease by "cutting" across it with a contrasting eyeshadow colour with little to no blending.

Whether your eyes are small, large, almond or hooded, a cut-crease will open them up for a beautiful, doe-eyed look. Additionally, the extra space created on the lids will offer a more extensive canvas to show off your favourite eyeshadows.

What's great about a cut-crease is that you can go super soft or really dramatic, depending on your mood.

In this section of the book, I am going to give you lots of techniques, hints and tips that you can use to create a variety of cut-crease eye looks from the traditional to the more vibrant and festive.

Originally a technique used in the 1960s by the likes of Twiggy, the cut-crease has grown in popularity and has taken over your social media walls and grids.

This look is so versatile and suits most eye shapes. The cut-crease looks complicated, yet it can be so easy to recreate whilst looking elaborate and sophisticated, taking your makeup to the next level. Your cut-crease can be created using any colours that take your fancy. Traditionally a cut-crease combines a lighter shade of eyeshadow on the lid and is cut with a darker shade across the crease of the eye, combined with a winged liquid liner and pair of false lashes for a truly glam look.

Easy Cut-crease

The classic cut-crease relies on two eye makeup staples you likely have in your makeup bag: eyeshadow colours and concealer.

1) Apply your concealer to your entire eye area

with a ring finger and massage into the skin for
an even application, let the concealer dry before
applying your chosen eyeshadow shades.

2) Your base eyeshadow will set the tone and vibe
for your makeup look. For this classic look,
you'll want to pick an eyeshadow colour that's
just a shade lighter than your skin tone and
apply this all over your lid starting from the
inner corner and blend up into the natural
crease.

3) Pick a dark contrasting colour, a warm brown is
traditionally used for a cut-crease. Use a slim
pencil crease brush and accurately draw a thin
line just above your natural crease, all the way
across from the middle of the lid and extend
out. Try looking down into the mirror when
applying your cutting. If you don't feel
confident drawing the shape, then try using a
plastic spoon as a template as this will give you
the perfect shape for cutting the crease. If you
are using the spoon as a template then I
recommend that you use a fluffier crease brush
to apply your contrast colour for a softer

application as you can always build this up later.
Sweep this colour back and forth across your
brow bone. Start slow and build up the
intensity in small circular motions to prevent
accidently lifting the colour or causing fallout.
You want the intensity along the underneath of
that brow bone.

4) You can choose to apply the same darker tone
across the lower lash line or leave it blank, it is
entirely up to you and depends on your desired
look.

5) Apply your favourite black liquid or gel liner
across your top lashes, extend and wing it out
for a sultry look.

6) Curl your lashes and apply lashings of black
mascara to the top and bottom lashes or apply
your choice of lashes for a more dramatic look.

Using powder eyeshadows in two colours makes
this look super easy to recreate, just remember to
make sure your cutting shade is a darker version of
the colour used on the lid for a beautiful contrast.
You can also cut the crease with concealer or

foundation for an even more dramatic take on the cut-crease. Carry out step one and apply your primer all over the lid but instead of applying a skin tone shade on the eyelid, go to step three and apply your warm brown cutting shade to create the new crease.

Using a thin concealer brush, apply concealer all over the eyelid. Start in the centre of the upper lash line, blend it up and out towards your natural crease and the outer and inner corner of the eyes, sweep the concealer outward and across towards the tail of the eyebrow to create a semi-circle

Don't forget to set your concealer or foundation with a translucent powder, then apply a cream or white colour over the top of the concealer to really amp up the contrast and create a striking look. This is the perfect opportunity to choose if you want a full cut-crease or if you are feeling brave and want to tackle the half cut crease.

Half Cut-crease

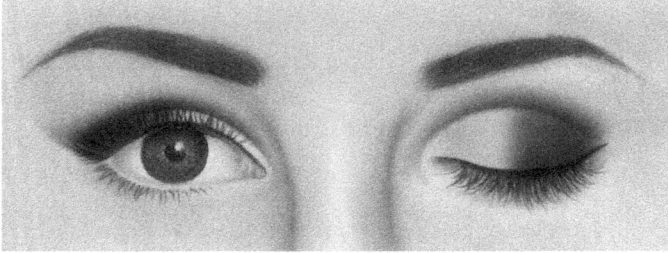

Once you feel like you have mastered the cut-crease and you are ready to take your makeup to the next level, then the half cut-crease is the next technique to try and is a great opportunity for experimenting with bold colours, metallics and glitter.

The main difference between the two cut-creases is for the half cut-crease, the colour above the cut-crease is extended down onto the lid and blended on the outer third of the eyelid extending inwards towards the middle and blended up and out to create a V-shape on the outer corner of the eye. This colour is blended into the crease, onto the outer corner of the eye and lower lash line. Much like the gradient smoky eye (see the Smoky Eyes chapter if you want to learn how to create a gradient smoky eye).

162

You will repeat the same steps as you did before to create the cut-crease except that after you have applied your concealer onto the lid and set it, you then use the same colour you used on the crease and blend this into the outer corner of the eye with a crease brush and blend it out. I recommend tracing this same colour onto your outer lower lash line for a coherent look.

If you want to use metallics or glitter products then I recommend that you apply them with your finger to the eyelids from the inner corner of the eye and towards the middle of the lid, make sure your crease remains glitter free and is well blended.

I recommend matching your glitter colour to that of the shadow above the crease, just make sure to use a slightly darker version of the glitter shade for the crease shade as this will create depth and give you a beautiful look.

You can also use neutral shades of glitter, for example a champagne tone, and a darker shade above on the crease for a beautiful bold look.

Apply your favourite winged eyeliner, mascara and choice of lashes.

Cut-crease Colours

If you have olive and darker skin tones then a purple cut crease will look especially good on you and is a perfect companion for people with greeny-blue, green or hazel eyes.

Feeling adventurous? Then try out a red cut-crease. This will look striking with dark blue, hazel or green eyes. Try applying a dark copper red if you are put off with the idea of using fire engine red.

A silver grey will highlight brown eyes beautifully but would also look amazing on light blue or grey eyes for a piercing modern result.

If you are looking for something fun and flirty for a night out then the pink cut-crease is for you and will make your blue eyes sparkle but the key is choosing the best pink shade to suit your eye colour. If you have light blue eyes use shades such as salmon or coral. Coral will look incredible on darker blue. If you have hazel or green eyes, a dusty metallic pink will really stand out.

A burgundy cut-crease looks great with all eye colours but particularly beautiful with dark blue or green eyes. Team with a burgundy lip for a bold look.

If you have hooded eyes, then the cut-crease is the perfect makeup look to try as it will make your eyes appear larger than normal. Make sure you follow the natural contour of the eye and blend upwards and outwards.

Recommended Tools

Please see the Eye Makeup Brushes Section for my recommendation of brush shapes to use when creating all of your eye makeup looks.

If you still feel a little apprehensive about your cut-crease placement then there are stencils available that will suit all eye shapes. They are a silicone shield that you can use to place over your eyelid, you then use a soft crease brush to draw round it to create your cut shape. Before spending any money, try using a plastic spoon first as you may find this will work perfectly for your eye shape.

Once you have mastered the cut-crease, your imagination and the colours you have in your makeup bag are your only limitations. Go wild and try out different colour combinations and different textures, such as metallics and glitter, and have fun creating your own unique looks.

Have a go at lining the edge between the light and the darker shade with a thin line of glitter for a fun glam look.

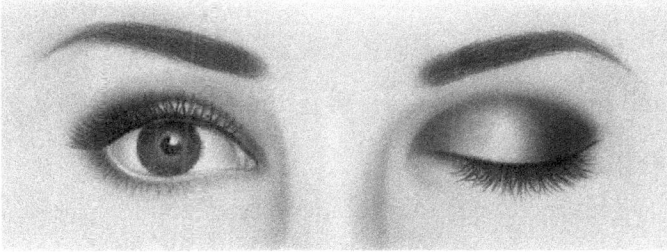

10. THE HALO EYE

The halo eye is a technique and a fairly recent trend that basically sandwiches a light-coloured eyeshadow, cream or foil in between a darker shadow on both sides and this is replicated both on the upper and lower eyelids.

Whether your eyes are small, large, almond, or hooded, a halo eye brings light to the center of the eye making your eyes appear larger, wider and rounder, and with a little tweaking will suit all eye shapes.

What's great about a halo eye, or spotlight eye as it sometimes known by, is that you can go soft or really dramatic depending on your mood. It can be done in any colour scheme and any finish so it can be tailored to suit all occasions.

In this section of the book are lots of techniques and tips that you can use to create your ideal halo eye look.

This technique may look complicated but believe me it is super easy to do, is so versatile and suits most eye shapes. It is incredibly flattering and dramatic yet soft, so you can really wear it at any time and it can be created using any colours that take your fancy.

Halo Eye Application Technique

You will need four eyeshadow shades in whatever colour choice you want. You could choose to contrast with your natural eye colour if you wished or you could even match the colours to your outfit, you just need to ensure that you have a light colour, a dark colour, a medium colour and a neutral.

- Prime your eyelids first, neutralise any discoloration redness, veins, etc, with a skin tone concealer or eyeshadow primer. Make sure you set this with translucent powder or a skin-toned powder to help make your colours more vibrant and your eye makeup last much longer. This can easily be applied with a finger or a concealer brush and set with a fluffy brush or powder puff.

- Apply a transition shade of shadow to the natural eye crease. A transition shade is a tone of eyeshadow that is one to two shades darker than your skin tone to help blend your colours out, however for a halo eye you want to keep this tone light as the focus is going to be on the lid and outer corner. Use a fluffy crease brush and a windscreen wiper motion to apply and blend. Remember the bigger the fluffy brush you use, the softer the result on the skin.

- Using a smaller crease brush apply a mid-tone of whatever colour scheme you have chosen to the inner and outer third of the eye. You want the colour on the inner third of the eye to be just as dark as the outer corner. Make sure you are leaving a neutral section in the centre of the eyelid above the pupil that does not have any product on it as this is where the light shade is going to be applied.

- Using the same small crease brush, use either a black or a darker shade of the same colour scheme and apply this on the outer corner of the eye and inner third of the eye using small circular motions. Blend into your medium shade using a fluffy brush to blend the two seamlessly together ensuring you leave that neutral zone in the centre of the eyelid without any product on it.

- This is the entire focal point of the halo makeup look, the pop of 'light' in the centre of the eyelid. You can either go in with a foil shadow using a finger to apply this to the eye for a smooth application or apply a bright bold pop of colour, white also works well. Apply this to the eyelid to add the light to the look. If you want something more dramatic and intense, apply a little bit of your concealer or the primer you used into the neutral part of the eyelid and blend it into the surrounding colour, then pat on your choice of colour over the top, this will help intensify your colours. Make sure you blend the edges of your 'light' colour into the inner and outer corners for a beautiful blended look.

- Repeat the same technique and use the same products along the lower lash line ensuring that the light shade lines up with the pupil. Use a pencil crease brush for a precise application.

- Apply a nude eyeliner to open up and brighten the eye or a black eyeliner to make the look more dramatic along your lower waterline. You may not need to use eyeliner with this look as we are creating a round eye. If we were apply a wing or a flick this will likely distort the overall shape of the eye.

- Apply a little bit of a highlighter or the same 'light' colour using a tiny pencil crease brush to apply to the inner corner of the eye to help open and brighten the eye up.

- Apply your mascara and false lashes if you choose too.

- Don't forget to groom those brows as a well-groomed brow makes a world of difference to any eye makeup but especially for one that is as bold as the halo eye, it will really finish the look.

I really like to use matte shades for the outer and inner thirds of the eye and hit that central spot of the eyelid with a shimmery, satin foil shadow applied with a finger for the best eye-catching results. You can also use the foiling technique and make any eyeshadow more intense by using a dampened brush (with setting spray) to apply for a better colour intensity.

When creating your halo eye, I recommend working within the same colour spectrum, for example if you were to apply a dark grey for the outer and inner third then I would use a light metallic grey or silver as the 'light' shade. But this is where you can get really creative and create some beautiful bright and colourful makeup.

Tips on Applying Your Halo Eye

- If you have a mono lid, I recommend avoiding using deep shades on the inner corner of the eye.

- If you have close-set eyes, avoid wearing contrasting colours as this can make your eyes appear closer, instead use colours of the same colour spectrum for a more flattering result.

- A halo eye can be tricky to master on a hooded eye but it is not impossible so keep trying. I recommend blending the colours ever so slightly above the natural eye crease so you can see the effects of the halo when the eye is open, use the taupe transition shade across the hood to minimise its effects.

- Always use an eye primer before applying any products to the eyelids as this will provide you with a better colour payoff and will last much longer without creasing and sliding off throughout the day.

- Think about the balance of your face. If you're using dark or bright colours on the eyes then choose to minimise the rest of your makeup to not overdo the look.

- Blending is an important aspect of creating a halo eye. Use larger fluffy brushes for the lighter colours and for applying shadows on large surface areas of the eyelid. When applying the darker shades or you want to have more concentrated intensity then use a smaller crease brush or blending brush to apply your makeup more precisely. This is a good brush shape to use for the lower lash line, inner corner of the eye and outer corner of the eye too.

- I always like to do any eye makeup first before applying any other products to the skin as this will allow for a quick and easy clean up, especially if you are using dark or glittery colours. Use a dampened brush to minimise the fallout.

Recommended Tools

Please see the Eye Makeup Brushes Section for my recommendations of brush shapes to use when creating all of your eye makeup looks.

I hope you enjoy playing with your halo eye creations. Have a go with creating your own foil shades with your shimmery eyeshadows and try adding some glitter to really glam up this look, perfect for a special occasion.

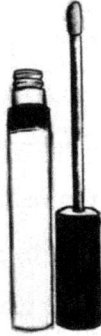

11. CONCEALER AND COLOUR CORRECTION/COLOUR THEORY

Concealer

Concealer is a type of makeup used to camouflage skin imperfections such as blemishes, pimples, acne, age spots, dark circles, uneven pigmentation and shadows. It can be used to contour by adding dimension to the body and face. Concealer is similar to foundation but tends to have more pigmentation and is a slightly thicker consistency than foundation. It is used to blend the imperfections into the surrounding skin tone.

Application Techniques

Concealer has lots of different uses, that is why there are so many different variations, formulas and colours available Understanding how and what they are best used for will help you in making your decision of which concealer you particularly need and want for your skin.

Two shades of concealer are useful to have as part of your everyday makeup kit.

- Shade One - should match the colour of your foundation and be used to cover general skin imperfections.
- Shade Two - for lighter skin tones, this should be a shade lighter than your foundation and used to hide unwanted shadows.
- Shade Two - for darker skin tones, this should be orange-toned to help disguise natural dark areas and hyperpigmentation.

Dark Under Eye Circles

When working with the under eye area, you want to

use a formula that is not too thick so that it can easily be blended into the skin and won't drag or settle into the fine lines under the eyes.

If you have particularly dark blue circles under the eye then colour correct this first using a peach colour corrector before applying your foundation and shade one concealer which will help camouflage those blue tones.

When working with any concealer you want to be working with the same undertone as your foundation and try not to go too light with the shade, ideally go half to one shade lighter than your skin tone to help brighten up those areas.

When applying concealer under the eye, make sure you are using a concealer the same colour as your foundation to help conceal any redness or purple hues that can be common along the lower lash line, and prevent enhancing dark circles.

Apply your concealer as an inverted triangle so the tip is pointing toward your cheek in shade one or lighter as this will help brighten up the entire centre of the face.

Another method is to apply a lighter shade of

concealer to the inner corner of the eye, down the side of the nose and to the outer corner of the eye at a 45-degree angle, this will help lift the eye area and make you look more awake and alert.

Less is always more when it comes to concealer and foundation. I always apply my foundation first, before any concealer, as this will cover up the majority of the imperfections I would want to fix with the concealer. I can then go in with a lighter hand and only use concealer in the areas that need further coverage. If any colour correction is required then apply it before foundation as the colour corrector you use may require concealing with a skin tone.

Spot/Acne/Pimple Camouflage

When concealing a spot, you want to use a thicker formula like a cream or stick to ensure the product adheres to the problem area. Ensure it is set well before applying any other product on top to prevent it lifting off. If it is particularly red then I recommend using a green colour corrector to counteract the redness, use a tiny pointed brush for direct application to apply the product on top of the pimple to prevent creating a halo effect around the pimple/spot and making it more obvious. Make sure you blend it well and then apply your shade one concealer over the top followed by foundation. Don't forget to set it with translucent powder.

Contour and Highlight

You can easily use a light reflective concealer to contour, define and highlight your eyes and lips.

- Apply your pencil or liquid concealer under the brow bone, concentrated under the natural arch of the brow and blend well. Apply a > shape in the inner corner of the eye, next to the tear duct, this will help the eye look wider and more awake. Concealer can also be used on the centre of the eyelid to add a natural highlight, just make sure it is well blended to create a natural highlight.
- Lips can be made to look plumper by drawing a V to define the cupids bow and extend up the philtrum. Make sure it is all well blended before applying your favourite lippy.

Types of Concealer

Cream:

- Thick consistency.
- Matte finish.
- Pimples.
- Blemishes.
- Dark under eye circles.

Body Stick/Panstick:

- Thick consistency.
- Matte finish.
- Blemishes.
- Camouflages veins, tattoos.

Stick:

- Great for on the go and for touch ups.
- Blemishes.
- Pimples/acne/spots.

Pencil:

- Thick consistency.

- Semi-matte finish.

- Good for drawing on highlights and contours.

Recommended Brushes and Tools

There are lots of different tools available to apply and blend concealers, including the applicators some concealers come with, like the pen, wand and pencil varieties, but these still need to be well blended into the skin.

Stipple Brush

This type of brush will give you a natural coverage and airbrush look and feel to the finish of your makeup. The brush deposits minimal product and as a result is great for covering up imperfections and scars in the skin. The coverage can be built up in thin layers by stippling and dabbing the brush across the surface of the skin. This brush is suited for cream and liquid foundations and concealers.

You can also get a smaller version of a stipple brush which is a great brush for buffing on concealer. I recommend using this type of brush for when you want to be covering a large textured surface with concealer to ensure you get a natural result.

Sponges

Latex sponges can provide a flawless streak free application and work really well with a dry skin as the sponge works best when it is slightly damp therefore adding moisture to the face, however this can weaken the coverage and pigment of the foundation. You never want to rub with a sponge as this will remove product, you are better off dabbing or rocking the sponge on the skin to distribute product. The sponge is best used for blending liquid foundation, concealer and contour as well as applying and removing excess powder.

Concealer Brushes

A concealer brush is used for applying cream and liquid concealer to the skin. The concealer brush looks similar to the flat eyeshadow brush but is usually slightly narrower and the dense shape makes it great for applying cream concealer. The fluffy crease brush is another great shape of brush perfect for blending and buffing concealer into the skin. Use a flat small concealer brush to apply concealer to small areas of the face and under the eye, and blend with a fluffy crease brush or a clean ring finger to help melt the product seamlessly into the skin. Do not forget to set all your concealer and foundation with a translucent powder to prolong their longevity and durability on the skin.

Colour Correction and Colour Theory

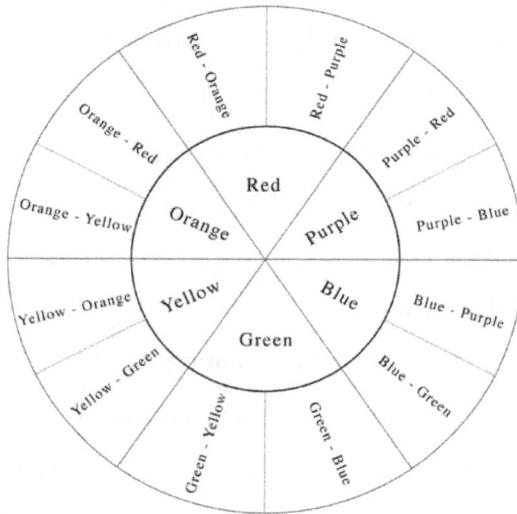

Colour corrector is very similar to concealer in consistency; however colour correctors tend to be highly pigmented and made up of colours like peach, yellow, pink and green. It is used for camouflaging skin imperfections like discoloration, uneven pigmentation, shadows, acne, burns, dark circles, tattoos and scarring.

Colour Theory

Colour correction can be used for a variety of camouflaging applications ranging from the simple concealment of dark under eye circles to the more extreme camouflage of scarring caused from various incidents including burns, tattoos, operations, cancers and accidents. In this guide, I am focusing more on the general everyday application of colour correcting like covering that pesky red pimple that has decided to rear its ugly head right before an important event or occasion that you have to get to.

Colour theory plays a major part when designing and applying any makeup. When colour correcting, you need to understand how colour can be affected by other colours. The main thing to be aware of when colour correcting is using colours that are opposite each other on the colour wheel as these colours will help neutralise one another.

Let me put this into terms of makeup colour correcting; green is opposite red on a colour wheel, therefore a green-based concealer can be used to neutralise unwanted redness in the skin such as rosacea, sunburn, spots and blemishes.

Purple is opposite yellow on the colour wheel and can be used to neutralise yellow tones in the skin. Lilac tones for fair skin and mauve for darker skin tones can be used to help neutralise unwanted yellow tones in the skin, in turn brightening the complexion.

On the market today you can easily pick up a concealer that already contains a colour corrector so you can buy a product that is specifically targeted to your needs, i.e. to brighten a complexion, to combat rosacea, pimples or to conceal dark eye circles or all of the above.

As a makeup artist, because I work with so many different clients, I have to be able to camouflage and conceal lots of skin tones so I need to provide a range of colours that can be tailored to suit my clients' needs in my kit. I have opted for a colour corrector palette instead of an individual product. I have a small palette of colour correctors that I can easily mix with neutral or skin tone concealers. I also use skin perfecting primers that colour correct and brighten the skin before any makeup products are applied.

Colours Used for Colour Correcting

Green (Mint to Dark Green)

Neutralises redness in the skin like rosacea, pimples and scars.

Purple (Lilac to Mauve)

Cancels out yellow tones, particularly good for Asian skin and brightening the complexion. Lilac should be used for fair skin and mauve tones for dark skin.

Pink/Rose

Brightens blue tones in a Caucasian skin.
Rose will neutralise green tones.

Peach/Orange

Neutralises blue and purple shades on medium/dark

skin tones and dark under eye shadows.

It can be mixed with a matching skin tone to cancel
out dark pigments on dark skin.

Yellow

Brightens purple or darker tones, great for olive and
tanned skin tones.

White and Neutral

Great to use as highlighters. Good for mixing with
the colour correctors to create paler versions and help
them blend into the skin to give a more natural result.
Apply a white mixed with matching skin tone to
cancel out dark brown areas on light skin.

Application Techniques

I have included a few common issues that may
require some colour correction, I could write an entire
book alone on colour correction for all skin ailments
but for the purpose of this book I have chosen to
include the most common issues that you are likely to
come across.

Hyperpigmentation/Age Spots

Hyperpigmentation is a common, usually harmless condition in which patches of skin become darker in colour than the normal surrounding skin. The most common form of skin hyperpigmentation is age or liver spots.

- The best colour to help disguise and neutralise a dark spot is a peach/orange tone. This should be applied before applying your matching skin tone foundation to help disguise the dark spots.

- Apply your choice of primer to your entre face or just to the problem areas if you wish.

- Using a colour corrector in an orange/peach shade suitable for your skin tone, use a flat concealer brush or your fingers to apply your product. I recommend putting the concealer onto the back of your hand first and lightly pick up the colour with your finger or brush and layer up the product onto the dark spot in a dabbing motion to gradually deposit colour to give a more natural result rather than applying a thick layer that will likely be difficult to blend into the skin.

- Use a pale peach for fair skins, medium peach for medium skins and darker peach tone for darker skins.

- Apply your choice of peach tone onto the dark spot and blend out the edges into the surrounding skin for a natural result.

- If your dark spots are not too dark then try using your skin tone concealer instead of the peach tone or try mixing the two together for a more muted peach tone. Buff onto the dark spot and layer up gradually for the most flattering result. Make sure you set it before applying your foundation.

- Apply your full coverage skin tone concealer over the top of the colour correction to help disguise the dark areas further if you feel you need to .

- Apply your choice of foundation in your skin tone over the top and set it all in place with translucent powder and setting spray.

Hypopigmentation

Hypopigmentation refers to patches of skin that are lighter than your overall skin tone. The most common of this is called vitiligo which is the complete loss of pigmentation. It can occur all over the body but often affects the face.

Before applying your skin tone foundation, apply your primer and a muted yellow-orange tone to the areas that have lost pigmentation, the darker the skin the more orange the tone needs to be. Apply the colour to the problem areas and blend over the edge to disguise, blend and soften the demarcation line. Set the colour correcting with a translucent powder and apply your favourite foundation shade and set with powder.

Rosacea

Rosacea is a skin condition that mainly affects the face and is most common amongst fair-skinned people. Rosacea can have a few different visual attributes such as superficial redness across the cheeks and nose. You may have broken capillaries across your cheeks although this tends to be a symptom amongst older people. Sometimes you can get tiny pink or red bumps that form on the skin causing the appearance of redness and can be quite sore. I am not a doctor and I am not diagnosing your skin problem but if you have rosacea I know that this can be of big concern to some people and can cause a lot of anxiety. There is no cure but with the right makeup application you can successfully cover up the redness and feel more confident in your skin.

- Apply a hydrating primer to the problem area to create a smooth base and help your makeup adhere and last much longer. You can use clean hands to apply your primer.
- Using an olive green cream concealer, apply lightly to the problem area. If it is a large surface area then I recommend using a sponge or stipple sponge. Buff the product lightly into the skin to prevent irritating the skin whilst maintaining a natural result.
- Apply a translucent powder with a fluffy powder brush and let the product sit for a minute or two. Check if redness is still visible

and if it is, apply another layer of that olive green. Once you are happy with the coverage of the redness, set with translucent powder.

- Apply your skin tone concealer over the top to neutralise the green and then you can apply your favourite foundation product. I suggest using a liquid or cream foundation to provide adequate coverage. Don't forget to set your base.

- If you skin already has a lot of colour, I would avoid applying blush. Instead, try applying a bronzer for a natural healthy warm glow.

I bet you never knew there was so much to consider when choosing and applying your makeup base. But once you know your own skin and what it needs, you will be able to choose and use the most suitable products effectively that are perfect for you and your skin.

How Lighting Affects the Colour of Makeup

Lighting is important for colour accuracy when applying your makeup. Without going into too much depth around the science behind how light affects makeup, this section aims to give you a brief overview of how different lighting conditions may affect your makeup application and appearance.

Have you ever tried on makeup in a store only to step outside and for it to be completely the wrong shade or look too heavy?

Chances are the makeup was applied under fluorescent or tungsten lighting which will affect how your skin and makeup looks when viewed outside. Makeup often looks heavier and warmer when applied in tungsten lighting (the lights like you have at home, for example). If your makeup is applied under fluorescent lights (like you have in your kitchen or bathroom and on most shop floors), when your makeup is viewed under natural light it may appear cooler and washed out.

As I am sure you already know the best light to apply your makeup in is daylight as this gives the truer representation of your makeup colours, textures and application technique. The natural light will show up any makeup mishaps or mismatches. Daylight is the best type of light to apply your makeup for an accurate application.

When working with my clients, I take into consideration the occasion and time of day the makeup is going to be viewed as this can alter the way I apply the makeup. If it is for a night out then I make more emphasis on the eyes and lips as this type of makeup is more likely to be viewed under artificial lighting, therefore it needs to be applied stronger.

When working on my brides, for example, they are likely to be viewed in all types of lighting as well as daylight so I always like to apply my makeup in as much natural light as possible. I will position myself in front of a window so my bride can look out into the light and I can see exactly what I am doing and check if the makeup is well applied, blended and that I am using the correct colours and intensity of the makeup for the skin. I then like to check my makeup in different lighting and through a camera lens, as I often find when I take an evidence photo sometimes my colours can seem a little paler than in person but because I have checked it, I can intensify colours where needed and I suggest that you do the same with your own makeup.

Invest in a light up mirror that has LED bulbs or promotes daylight as a feature for the most accurate results for your makeup application.

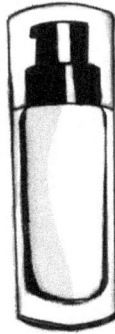

12. FOUNDATION

There are so many foundations out there on the
market, different tones, colours, textures and finishes,
it is going to be a little bit of trial and error until you
find one that you and your skin actually like.
Hopefully, this guide will help you towards choosing
your suitable foundation.

Why Do We Wear Foundation?

- To give the skin an even appearance.
- Achieve a healthy glow.

- Cover discoloration and uneven pigmentation.

- Protect skin from the environment.

- To hide dark circles and bags under the eyes.

- Even out blemishes and hide scars.

- Disguise effects of ageing on the skin, adding tone.

- A base for the rest of the makeup to stick to.

- To add depth and definition to the face.

- Make the wearer feel more confident in their own skin.

We strive to create a base that is flawless, radiant and long-lasting yet convincing enough to pass off as natural skin.

Your skin type is a really important thing to consider when choosing a suitable foundation, you also have to take into consideration your skin texture and what finish of foundation you want for your face as well as choosing a suitable colour to suit your skin tone.

Tinted Moisturiser

Technically this is not a foundation as it does not

offer much coverage, however it is great for enhancing a suntan or for use on a clear complexion skin. Tinted moisturiser is also good as a base for males as its finish is so sheer and light whilst adding a little bit of colour. I like to produce my own tinted moisturiser using my favourite moisturiser and a little bit of concealer or liquid foundation mixed in and I like to wear this on days when I just want a little something on the skin.

Liquid Foundation (Oil in Water)

Liquid foundation is available in different formulations of oil and water and is suitable for all the different skin types. This type of foundation allows the skin's natural glow to show through and is personally one of my favourites to use.

A liquid formula is non-sticky and can easily be mixed together to create exact skin matches and does not accentuate lines and pores, however some formulas can dry up to three shades darker and it has a short working time as it will dry before it has been set, so it needs to be applied swiftly and effectively. I do not recommend applying liquid foundations with your fingers as the heat from your hands can also affect the overall colour of the makeup finish. That being said, I love using liquid foundations on my own face as I really like the finish on the skin.

Cream Foundation

Cream foundations are easier to apply than a liquid formula as cream does not dry until it is set with powder, therefore it is easier to blend. There is no colour change with a cream foundation and it gives a full coverage so is perfect for photographic work.

Cream formulas are suitable for all skin types but especially good for a drier skin. This formula can be applied lightly, mixed with a moisturiser or applied to give a full coverage so it is very versatile and is the staple in most makeup artists kits and the foundation of choice for media makeup artists as they look good on camera.

A cream foundation, if unpowdered, gives a glossy finish to the skin but can be easily transferred or slip during hot weather or shoots so must be powdered to set them in place.

All-in-one Foundation (Powder and Foundation)

Easily applied with a damp sponge this formula dries to a matte finish that is very durable and

gives great coverage. It is convenient and quick as it does not need to be set, making it

perfect for touch ups on film sets. On the whole, it is good for an oily skin and use

in hot climates as it dries on the skin, therefore it is not suitable for a dry skin type. Because of its high powder content, it needs to be worked with quickly and effectively.

Mousse Foundation

Mousse foundation gives a minimal coverage, but it can be built up like a liquid foundation for a little extra coverage.

A mousse formula is easily blended but has to be applied quickly before its volume diminishes

and it does have a tendency to change colour when dry. I used to wear this type of formula in my teenage years (you know the one!) and I found not only would it change colour when dried, it also used to cling to the drier areas of the face and would end up looking patchy as soon as I left the house. This formula is great for a young skin that needs a light coverage but it is not a formula I have ever used on or recommended to any of my clients.

Airbrush Foundation

Airbrush foundations come in a variety of formulas and finishes, including aqua-based, alcohol-based and silicone. These are thin liquids that are applied through an airbrush and compressor or aerosol. I absolutely love airbrush foundations and it is what I have chosen to specialise in as a makeup artist. I exclusively use these for all my clients as they are so versatile, offer fantastic coverage and can be tailored to suit any skin type and tone quickly and easily. Because the liquids are so sheer, it can be built up in layers so I can offer my clients anything from a sheer finish to an opaque finish that will cover a black tattoo.

I personally love a silicone-based foundation as I find them to be the most durable, workable and they give a radiant flawless finish that is waterproof and that I love so much I use it on my own skin. I find the alcohol and aqua based formulas dry so fast that it does not give you any working time to blend if needed.

Gel Foundation

One of the newest additions to the foundation family, gel foundation is a lighter alternative to liquid foundation for a translucent finish. Colour pigments are suspended in a gel formulation

that glides on easily and absorbs well. The effect is very natural and sheer. It is excellent for

adding enhancement to tanned skin, however it wears off easily and can cause dryness

on sensitive skins.

Grease Foundations/Panstick

You may not necessarily come across this type of makeup in your local health and beauty retail shop due to it being designed for the stage, however I wanted to mention it as you may want to get some for your panto, production or Halloween party. This type of foundation provides a heavy coverage and is great for character makeups when there is lots of shading involved. It can be purchased in palettes or sticks and has a greater density of pigment than everyday foundation products. Grease based products need plenty of powdering to set and is not recommended for everyday use due to the heavy finish of the product.

Pancake Foundation

Used mainly for body makeup and where a flat look is required as on bald heads. Applied wet, pancake dries quickly to a matte finish which can be buffed with a cloth to produce a natural looking sheen. Pancake is long-lasting and durable but can be quite drying to the skin. This is another type of foundation you are unlikely to see in your local health and beauty retailer but again is worth mentioning as it has its uses.

Camouflage Foundation (Dermacolor)

This type of foundation is very highly pigmented and is designed to cover scars, birthmarks and burns, but is also useful to cover unwanted freckles, liver spots, beard shadow and tattoos. It is predominantly used for TV and film work but also for NHS patients. Due to it being water resistant, it is long-wearing. This foundation gives an excellent opaque coverage without the look of a heavy application. It can be layered up and mixed together to create custom shades. A Dermacolor palette is a staple in most makeup artists' kits.

FINISHES

You are likely to find these terms when talking about foundation finishes and textures on the product packaging so it's a good idea to familiarise yourself with these terms and what they mean to you so you can make an informed decision of the type of finish you would like for your skin. I personally like a dewy, satin finish as I feel it gives the most radiant, natural finish.

Demi-matte/Semi-matte/Satin/Velvet

These terms all mean the same type of finish and all give a flawless coverage with a slightly matte and light reflective finish. This type of finish is suitable for all skin types but due to being a full coverage, I would recommend it for skin with blemishes.

Dewy/Sheer

This type of finish gives a natural wet look to the skin, but without looking too oily due to most of these products being made of silicones, which give the appearance of a soft natural finish. This type of foundation does not offer a flawless coverage so it is more suitable for someone with a clearer complexion, however it can be used on any skin type.

Light Diffusing/Pore and Line Minimising/Light Reflective

These terms all mean the same type of finish and all give a light reflective, youthful glow, perfect for counteracting the effects of ageing on the skin and on a younger skin for creating a dewy, glowing finish. These products contain pigments that reflect the light off the skin so are good for disguising blemishes, thin lines, wrinkles and pores.

Matte/Oil Free

As this product does not contain any oil, it has a short working time so needs to be applied swiftly as it dries very quickly. This type of finish creates a very flat look that does not reflect the light. It is great for an oily skin as it stays shine free but can appear heavy on the surface of the skin. I don't tend to use completely matte formulas as I find them too flat on the skin and it does not look as natural as a light reflective finish. They are really great for doing period makeup so I do have them in my professional kit for photoshoots.

Oil Based

This type of formula offers good coverage but can appear heavier than other finishes. This type of formula adds moisture to the skin, so it is really good for a dry flaky skin, however it is not suitable for an oily skin type.

A non-comedogenic formula does not clog pores and is particularly good for an oily skin.

Maximum Cover/Total Cover/Opaque

These terms all mean the same thing when it comes

to the coverage of the foundation. An opaque coverage will disguise most imperfections and is suitable for all skin types, however it can have a heavier and flatter appearance on the skin.

UV Filters/SPF

Foundations that contain Sun Protective Factor (SPF) is more about the formula ingredients rather than the actual look and finish of the foundation on the skin. You can get foundations with SPF that are sheer, matte, light reflective, full coverage, etc. These types of foundations tend to be good for all skin types depending on their overall finish and great to use during the summer months and hotter climates. However, I do not recommend it for brides or models due to it causing flashbacks in professional photographs.

Pearlised

A pearlised foundation can be used on its own to create a wet look finish or, as I like to use it, as a highlighter when worn under, over or mixed in with another foundation. It adds a subtle shimmer to your complexion and looks great on youthful skin. Don't forget that foundations with shimmery finishes can create the same effect as SPF formulas causing problems with lighting on screen and photographs.

FINDING YOUR SKIN TONE

So now you have chosen the type and finish of the foundation. Like that wasn't hard enough, you now need to choose the colour and tone of your foundation to suit your skin tone.

Undertones

Firstly, we need to look at the undertones that are found within the skin so we can make an informed decision on whether we are warm, cool or neutral-toned when choosing our foundation shade. Most people have either yellow or pink undertones.

When choosing a foundation, you must take into account your skin tone to ensure that you choose the perfect match for your skin to prevent discolouring the skin by oversaturating it in too much yellow or pink, as this can look odd on the skin.

To identify the undertone of your skin, the best trick I find is to look at the underside of your wrist and focus on the veins. If they appear to be more blue then you have pink cool undertones. If the veins appear to be more green then you have yellow or golden warm undertones. Not everyone is just one or the other, sometimes both undertones will be evident and this would be considered to be neutral so you can choose to play one against the other by using shades or correctors that include or exclude your undertone.

Another way to identify your undertone is to look at your face in the mirror under natural daylight with no makeup on. If your skin appears to be more golden then it has yellow warm undertones, if your face appears to be more pink-beige then you have pink cool undertones.

Darker skin colours tend to be predominantly made up of golden, warmer yellowy undertones.

By identifying your undertone you have also identified whether you are warm, cool or neutral-toned so now when you are choosing your foundation you can look for skin shades that are either warm, cool or neutral.

Three Stripe Test (Testing Your Chosen Tones)

You now need to choose a suitable colour and tone of foundation; I like to do this by doing the three stripe test.

Choose three foundation shades you think are close to your skin tone that have your warm or cool undertone. Apply three stripes with your finger or a brush to the jawline and down the neck and on the forehead. I also like to put three spots on the chest to really ensure I am choosing the correct shade as the chest tends to catch more sun than the neck and if you wear face makeup daily, I find the face tends to be a lighter colour so, I always like to check these three areas to ensure the foundation is not going to look too light or dark on the skin. Whichever shade melts into the skin with little detection is your perfect colour but you need to make sure that it's undetectable in all three areas to ensure it is your perfect match.

Sometimes you may have to mix a couple of

shades together to achieve your correct skin tone, however there are so many foundations on the market you should have no problem choosing your correct colour.

In my personal kit, I like to have at least two different colour foundations but made with the same undertone and I recommend you do the same as our skin changes colour during the seasons. You may find in winter that your skin is slightly paler and in the summer it is likely to be warmer, so I like to mix my foundations to create my perfect shade to transition through the seasons with.

Top tip - make sure when trying out foundation colours that you look at them under natural daylight if possible and not just under the florescent lights in the retail shop as this will affect the colour of the foundation. A lot of people have told me they tried the foundation on and liked it in the store but when they got home it was completely the wrong colour, and once you open a foundation you cannot return it so it could be a costly mistake.

APPLYING YOUR FOUNDATION

There are many techniques and tools used for the application of foundation. The decision of what tool or technique is best for applying your foundation is the combination of personal choice and the desired finish.

In this section you will find the various application methods for your foundation.

Natural Sponge Method

The sponge must be damp to make it pliable, then it can be used to apply any foundation with a press and roll motion. It can produce a very light to full coverage. The texture of the natural sponge emulates the pores of the skin so the finish is very natural no matter how heavy it is applied.

Fingers

You would have heard me say earlier not to use your fingers when applying a liquid foundation. This is true but in some cases I like to use a sterilised ring finger to blend creams, especially a cream concealer under the eye area as the warmth of the finger helps blend the product into skin unlike a cold makeup brush.

Theatrical makeup artists use their fingers to blend wax foundations, as warmth from fingers will help to soften the wax formulas.

Blending with the fingers is not a readily acceptable method of application for professionals

Because fingers may be cold, may drag the skin and it's not hygienic, but like I said, it does have its uses and on your own face you can apply your foundation however you wish.

Painting Method

Use a foundation brush that is at least an inch wide and soft yet firm to paint on products for a flawless finish. The brush needs to remain quite dry during application to avoid brush

strokes and streaking. I don't personally like to use a foundation brush; I prefer to use a kabuki or stipple brush which I refer to as a fibre optic brush when applying my foundation.

Using a kabuki brush, which is a wide, full, soft brush that is cut flat, the foundation is applied by swirling the brush over the face to create a blanket coverage that is buffed into the skin to produce a more natural result than a foundation paint brush. This type of method works particularly well with cream and liquid foundations but again the brush must remain relatively dry to avoid streaking.

Wedge/Flat Sponge Method

When I was training a few years ago now I used to solely use latex wedge sponges as they were considered to be disposable. They're not great for the environment though but I used to do so many makeups per day, every week, I would not have time to thoroughly clean and dry a foundation brush between each lesson. I now only use brushes, but sponges seem to have made a big come back with the introduction of beauty blenders being sold in most stores now.

The shape of the wedge sponge or beauty blender is good for working around the eyes and nose. The sponge can be used wet or dry depending on the effect you would like to achieve. When using a sponge to roll, press and dab on the foundation, use a light hand to prevent the sponge from lifting off the foundation or leaving unsightly streaks on the base before the foundation is set with powder.

Tips on Applying Your Foundation

- Apply your foundation before any concealer as most imperfections and discolourations will be covered by the foundation.

- Foundation can be applied all over the face if you want a fuller coverage, or for a more natural look it can just be applied where it is needed. If you are looking for a more natural result then I recommend not applying too much foundation on the nose.

- Apply your foundation to the centre of the face and blend outwards towards the hairline and down the neck too. Make sure you do not get foundation in the hair.

- When blending your foundation down the neck, make sure this is well blended so you don't look you have on a foundation mask.

- Foundation will highlight wrinkles so make

sure it is well blended into the skin in the areas more prone to lines, like around the eyes. This is where I like to use a warm ring finger to dab the product and melt it into the skin.

- You can apply foundation to the lips as well, so you are able to correct or enhance the lip shape. This is a good idea if you know you are going to alter the shape of the lip, however I find foundation can actually alter the colour of the lipstick and also dry out the lip. I prefer to apply a lip balm whilst I do the foundation so when I come to do the lips they are nicely hydrated.

- If you have a suntan, or perhaps want the appearance of one, make sure you use a bronzer or a tanning product rather than try to use a foundation to create the effect as this will just look unsightly.

- Always do your eye makeup before your base as this saves time in cleaning up any eyeshadow fallout and then you can use the base to help neaten up any rough edges that may have happened during the application.

- Always make sure you conceal the eye area and set it as this will help prolong the longevity of your eye makeup and give you a neutral base to work on.

- Always use downwards strokes when applying any formulation of foundation to prevent the downy hairs on the face from lifting and becoming noticeable on the skin.

- If minor imperfections are still visible after an application of foundation then don't be afraid to apply another light layer to that area using a brush or tapping a finger to help blend and cover a small area.

- Never use one thick layer of foundation to cover up skin problems as this will be very hard to blend and to achieve a natural result.

- Foundation should be left to settle into the skin as the natural oils from the skin will soften the makeup and further blend the application. Make sure you view your makeup under natural light.

- Make sure you set your foundation with a pressed, loose or translucent powder to prolong the makeup's longevity and to help blend further powder products, such as blush, bronzer and contour.

- Always apply powder to powder and cream/liquid to cream/liquid, for example if you are using a powder blusher, you want to make sure you have set your foundation and concealer to prevent the blush from grabbing to an area and therefore becoming impossible to blend. You do not want to set your foundation if you intend to use another cream/liquid product like blush or contour as this could cause the product to dry out and appear flaky on the skin.

- Setting spray can be applied to the face after you have applied your primer but before the foundation and then applied again over the foundation to help your makeup last much longer.

Freckles

I am in no way saying freckles are a problem to get rid of, in fact far from it, I just love to see freckles, but some people may want to minimise their appearance. In which case you want to choose a foundation with a medium to full coverage and choose a colour ever so slightly darker than your natural skin tone, but lighter than your freckles to help camouflage them into the skin.

FOUNDATION BRUSHES

Have you ever wondered what all those different shapes and sizes of foundation brush actually do and can be used for?

Brushes come in all different shapes and sizes, some are flat and stiff, round and soft, angled or pointed and they come in different densities, but they all do the same job: apply your foundation. They create different finishes and effects. I am going to explain to you the types of foundation brush and what they can and should be used for and how.

Stipple Brush

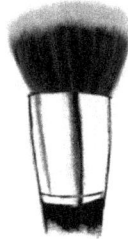

This type of brush will give you a natural coverage and airbrush look and feel to the finish of your makeup. The brush deposits minimal product and as a result is great for covering up imperfections and scars in the skin. The coverage can be built up in thin layers by stippling and dabbing the brush across the surface of the skin. This brush is suited for cream and liquid foundations.

I like to use a stipple brush on my own face as this allows me to buff the foundation into the skin rather than painting on a thick layer like a flat brush does. The stipple brush gives me a sheer coverage which can be built up to provide fuller coverage where needed but gives a more natural finish to the makeup.

Buffer Brush

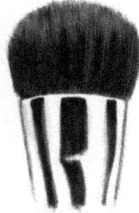

A buffer brush is made of densely packed hairs which create a firm texture but is also soft to the touch. This type of brush will give a sheer light coverage that, again, can be built up like the stipple brush by buffing and stippling the brush across the surface of the skin. This type of brush is not suitable for a dry skin type as the buffing motion acts like a mild exfoliate and will accentuate dry and flaky skin. This type of brush is best used for creams, liquids and powder foundations.

Flat Brush

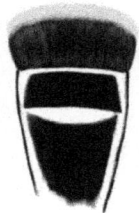

This is my least favourite brush to use for applying foundation as it gives a heavy coverage and can often leave streaks if not worked into the skin enough. I find I have to buff or stipple over the top to ensure a flawless coverage so I might as well just use a stipple or buffer brush in the first place, saving me time having to clean unnecessary brushes. The flat brush does have its uses and I like to use a smaller version of a flat brush to apply my concealer under and around the eye and nose, and then use a rounder fluffier brush to buff this into the skin. This brush is best used for cream and liquid foundations and concealer.

Pointed Brush

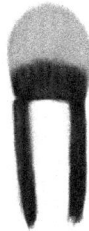

A pointed tapered brush is used to apply foundation and concealer more precisely around the eye area and the nose. I particularly use this brush for concealing and getting foundation blended to smaller areas on the face. This type of brush works well with creams and liquids just like the flat brush.

Kabuki Brush

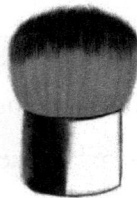

A kabuki brush is a short dense bristled brush with a short fat handle. This type of brush deposits more product than the previous brushes and will give a full coverage quickly. It is perfect for using with cream, liquid, powders and mineral powders. This brush can be used for quick effective application of a foundation base as it can be buffed into the skin and blended well. I personally use one of these brushes to apply my own foundation if I'm using a stipple brush.

Sponges

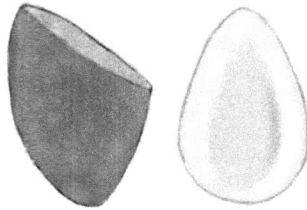

Latex sponges can provide a flawless streak free application and work really well with a dry skin as the sponge works best when it is slightly damp therefore adding moisture to the face, however this can weaken the coverage and pigment of the foundation. You never want to rub with a sponge as this will remove product, you are better off dabbing or rocking the sponge on the skin to distribute product. The sponge is best used for blending liquid foundation, concealer and contour as well as applying and removing excess powder.

A silicone sponge, although it looks like an insert from a high heeled shoe, is used to apply foundation. A silicone sponge is more environmentally friendly than a latex sponge and as they are not porous, they don't soak up the foundation like a latex sponge so there is less wasted product and every drop of foundation is applied to the face. However, due to the smooth texture of the sponge, it just spreads the product around giving a medium to full coverage which some people may like but if you are looking for something more natural or sheerer then this sponge is not for you. Whereas the latex sponge is soft and pliable so it allows for flawless blending into the skin.

Oval Brush

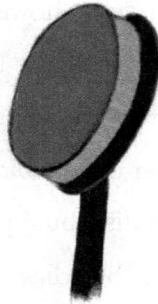

The oval shape brush is still fairly new to the industry and, as a makeup artist, I have not had much experience with them. The size and shape of the oval brush allows for quick and easy application, the bristles although soft are quite dense and act like a mini kabuki brush.

You may have come across a brush that has a slight well or hole in the middle of the bristles, this is for the foundation to be put in and helps distribute the right amount of product onto the skin.

So, it is safe to say there are lots of different brushes and sponges available for you to use for applying your foundation. I hope you have found this chapter useful and that it will help you choose the right tool and technique for you and your desired foundation application.

Hopefully, you now know how to choose and apply your most suitable foundation type, finish and shade by understanding your skin's undertone. You will be able to conceal and colour correct any minor skin issues that you may have and get your skin prepped and primed and ready for your makeup application.

13. CONTOURING

I know contouring sounds scary due to it being associated with on trend reality TV celebrities, but it really is not hard and it does not need to be so overpowering. A lot of the contouring you would have seen in magazines and on TV was designed to be seen under specific lighting and shot at multiple camera angles but in true life it would look unnatural.

I am going to give you all the knowledge and techniques you need, so you can learn how to define your facial features naturally.

Contouring is, or was, about changing and enhancing the shape of the face with makeup. This trend originated in the drag community and only in the past few years has the beauty industry adopted it and it's now seen as a standard part of a makeup regime. I am not here to tell you to forget about contouring, but I am going to teach you ways you can do it effectively, naturally and quickly so you can embrace your natural face shape.

Contouring is about creating dimension and depth to make facial features more or less pronounced using shade, shadow and darkness, i.e. contour makes things look smaller, thinner, deeper and removes harsh angles and minimises features, whereas highlighter makes things look bigger, maximises features and makes angles more pronounced and enhanced, and brings facial features forward. Both contour and highlighter together add depth, dimension and contours to the face and its features.

When it comes to contouring, the idea is to try and create, enhance or change a face shape to resemble the most attractive, symmetrical and aesthetically pleasing shape: the oval.

When I was teaching my students the art of contouring, I used to draw the geometric shape on the board and we would discuss how we would change each shape to resemble an oval. An easy way to do this is if you think about the face being a generic shape, like a square, for example, or a diamond, then the purpose of contour is to remove or minimise the angles, i.e. the corners of the shape, and make the width narrower by shading down the sides to make the face look less angular and softer like an oval, or in the case of a rectangle, it's about shortening the length by shading the ends.

That being said, there is nothing wrong with your face shape and when I'm working with my clients and on my own face, I don't try to make the face into an oval. I work on enhancing the features of the face in front of me, e.g. I like to define my cheekbones and minimise my jawline. I don't like to contour people's noses unless I am asked specifically to do so as I am a big believer in working with what I have got and celebrating individuality.

CONTOUR PRODUCTS

Makeup retailers will tell you that you must use/purchase a contour palette, the latest contour stick and only use products that are designed just for contouring but this is not the case. You can use products you probably already have in your makeup bag including foundation, concealer and eyeshadows, to contour with. Unless, of course, you want the latest strobe cream then, of course, go for it. Who does not love buying new makeup – I know I do.

Contouring is now seen as a standard part of every makeup regime whether it's contoured, highlighted, strobed or baked. I am going to tell you all about contour and highlight products and the effects that they have on the skin. I am going to teach you ways in which you can contour your face effectively, naturally and quickly so you can embrace your natural face shape.

Contouring used to be about changing the entire shape of your face with makeup but now it is more about embracing your natural shape and creating dimension and depth.

When choosing your contour shade you want to use a shade one to two shades darker than your natural skin tone, any darker and it may start looking unnatural and become difficult to blend effectively.

For modern contouring, you want to work with your natural undertones, skin tones and skin type when choosing your contour and highlight products and colours. When choosing a contour shade, always make sure your product is matte. Bronzer is not the same thing as contour as they are often made with illuminating particles and come off too dark and orange tinted, instead opt to use taupe-nude tones for a more natural result. You are trying to create depth and shadow so you need a product that gives the illusion of shadows, not a fake tan.

Bronzer is for adding a sun-kissed glow to the face like you have spent all day sitting on an exotic island, and it is applied to the face where the light would naturally hit, on the chin, nose, forehead and cheeks.

There are literally hundreds of contour and highlight products on the market so I have chosen to talk more about the formulas and colours rather than the physical products, so you can make an informed decision on the best product that will work for you and your skin.

Foundation/Cream

Foundation and concealer cream products are my favourite products to use when contouring as they're really easy to use and easily accessible in most supermarkets and retail outlets. This formula blends and melts into the skin and looks really natural once it has been set, it can also easily be enhanced with powder if needed for a stronger contour. Most people will have a couple of shades of foundation in their kit or they should have, as throughout the year our skin changes colour therefore so should our base.

Using a shade only a couple of shades darker than your normal foundation means that it is easily blended, mistakes can be hidden, and it can be built up to achieve your ideal contour shade.

Foundation or cream contour formulas always require setting either with a translucent powder, pressed powder or powder contour product. You cannot apply a cream formula on top of powder so make sure if your base is cream or liquid that you set your makeup after you have contoured.

This type of formula is suitable for mature skin and dry skin types and if you find makeup tends to settle into your fine lines or makes pores appear larger then try using a cream based formula instead of the powdery versions.

Powder

Powder formulas are perfect for oily skin types and younger poreless skin and can give an almost airbrushed effect with a matte velvety finish. If you are going to use a powder contour, make sure your base is set well before applying your powder contour to prevent your product from sticking and being unblendable. Powders are easily blended together and longer lasting than cream products but require more application technique. When it comes to using powder contour products, you can buy contour palettes or you can just use nude-taupe, brown-grey eyeshadows, as long as they have a matte finish.

Make sure you are working with your undertones when choosing your contour shade. If you are cool-toned ensure you are using cool tones for your contour shade, e.g. brown-greys. If you have warm undertones then you want to use warmer tones but make sure you don't go too orange otherwise it will look unnatural and could look overdone.

Application Techniques Tips

- If you use a brush with blunt bristles like a kabuki or square-ended brush then you will create a sharper contour. This is good for applying your contour guidelines. A fluffy brush like a contour brush that is angled or a large crease brush will diffuse the product giving you a much softer contour, this shape brush is perfect for blending.

- Make sure you use a smaller brush when contouring the nose and smaller features on the face.

- Use different brushes for application and blending, do not blend your highlight with the same contour brush as this will just muddy up your colours.

- If you are using a beauty blender or sponge to blend in your cream products then make sure that it is not too wet to avoid just pushing the products around the face.

- A good tip to really enhance and finish your contour is to highlight it with a lighter concealer or illuminating product.

- For those of you with a less steady hand or are perhaps less savvy or you may be nervous about contouring, start off with a foundation and concealer sticks and you can't go wrong.

- When contouring your cheekbones, apply your product slightly onto the cheekbone as this will help elevate and lift the face.

- Don't suck in your cheeks (fish face). This is an old technique, however if you must, please make sure you taper your contour. The intensity of the shade should be nearer the ears and taper out (get thinner) towards the center of the face, don't contour the cheek past the natural pupil (looking straight ahead) or risk looking overdone.

- If you want a stronger look then use both cream and powder products and remember to apply cream on cream and powder on powder.

HIGHLIGHT PRODUCTS

Highlighting has become such a huge thing in the makeup industry and when it is done right, it can look amazing, like you have been lit from within and it gives a beautiful youthful glow. But when it is done incorrectly, it can be disastrous. Too glittery, you end up looking like a disco ball, too pale and you end up looking sickly.

I am going to give you all the knowledge and techniques you need to highlight your facial features naturally.

Highlighter, aka strobing, can be used to make makeup look dewy or add a little sparkle to brighten up a face, as if it has just been freshly moisturised. It is not supposed to be shiny and glittery, it's not really designed to be seen from space either. It is supposed to give you the lit from within glow. Photographers will back me up with this, overly shiny, glittery products cause flashback in photographs so it is best to avoid or limit the use of them. If you intend to have your picture taken, for example at your wedding, instead choose to use HD (high definition) ready products which are designed to be seen on camera.

There are so many highlighting products available on the market, such as powders, liquid drops and creams, I am going to concentrate more on the formulas, tones and the effects that they have on the skin so you can choose the right formula, tone and finish that is perfect for you.

Highlighting a contour can be as simple as using the same product you used to contour with, like your cream or powder, but if it is one to two shades lighter than your contour shade, this will help add definition and enhance any shadow. It will make things look bigger, maximise and enhance and make your angles more prominent and bring the highlighted parts of the face forward.

Highlight is the ying to the yang of contouring, you don't tend to do one without the other. That being said, the strobing trend is all about adding light to the face without the contouring element. It is a simple technique that involves illuminating particular areas of the face to brighten, awaken and create a healthy, youthful look.

However, when it comes to choosing your highlighter or strobing product, it is not a one colour suits all scenario. Unfortunately, you still need to be working with your skin tone when choosing your ideal highlighter shade.

Skin Tones

Fair Skin

If you have pale, fair, cool-toned skin then you want to use highlighters that are pearlescent or iridescent. Opt for cooler shades like pearl, champagne, silver, light pink or peach tones and avoid deep shades like bronzer and copper as this may look a little garish and fake on the skin. We are going for the lit from within glow not a nuclear fallout glow.

Medium/Warm Skin

If you have a warmer/medium skin tone, you want to stay away from cool tones like pearl, silver and pink as these will look too frosty and harsh with your complexion. Instead, choose a highlighter with gold-bronze, darker peach or golden undertones. You can still wear iridescent shades just make sure that they are of a warmer tone.

Dark Skin

If you have a dark skin tone, you want to also stay away from cool tones like pearl, silver and pink as these will look too frosty and could appear ashy with your complexion. Instead, choose a highlighter with a higher pigmentation with rose-gold, bronze, copper or deep gold undertones. Steer clear of opalescent, frosty shades and too much shimmer as these can come across quite grey on a dark skin.

Not all highlighter products do the same thing, some will help you add a beautiful subtle sheen to the skin whilst others will add more glimmer, glitter and glamour or will provide you with an out of this world holographic, rainbow and chrome effect.

I am not here to judge and I want people to have fun with their makeup but perhaps these more artistic colours would be better suited for special occasions and not necessarily an essential part to your everyday makeup.

Cream

Cream based highlighters, also known as strobing creams, can be worn under your foundation base to act as an illuminating primer. This can give a really lovely sheen to the skin and brighten up any complexion. This product can also be applied on top of your base before the base is set, on the highlighting points suitable for your face shape and applied to other parts of the body. Cream formulas contain a lot of pigment compared to other highlighting products so they are a good choice if you are looking for more of a glam, powerful look. Blend with your finger for a more natural finish.

Liquid/Drops

Liquid highlighters are incredibly pigmented and a

little goes a long way. They can be applied under your base or mixed with your choice of foundation to add a glow to your skin. When working with this type of formula it needs to be worked with quickly as it dries fast and is best used with a confident hand. You can add this product on top of your base but I prefer to use liquid formulas mixed into foundations to create a glow.

Stick

Highlighter in a stick format is easy to use and can literally be drawn onto the facial high points and easily blended with a brush or finger. This product is great swiped on your eyelids to create an instant brightening effect.

A great product for a newbie strober.

Powder

This formula is the most common and is the softest way to accentuate your features and create an overall fresh-looking face. I have powder highlighters as part of my professional and personal makeup kit. Powder highlighter is like a pressed powder or compact except it has an illuminating finish. This product is best applied with a fan brush and last as part of your makeup routine after the base has been set. Apply this product to your cupid's bow to enhance your pout. Apply powder highlighter to the inner corner of the eyes to open them up and wake up your makeup.

Brick Highlighter

You would have seen this product everywhere; most makeup brands have their own version. It is a pressed powder made up of various sections of different tones of highlighter which can individually be selected and applied to the face or you can mix all tones together to form your own highlight colour or apply all of them at once to create a layered effect. This type of product comes in so many variations of colours, even rainbow, chrome, etc. I would recommend a natural look to work with your skin tone when choosing your brick highlighter.

Application Technique Tips

- Mix in a few drops of liquid highlighter with

your moisturiser or foundation for an all over radiant glow.

- Apply highlighter to the inner corner of the eyes, under the brow bone and to the center of eyelids for an instant eye brightening lift.

- When highlighting your cheekbones, blend right up to the temples to help lift the face.

- Apply highlighter to your cupid's bow and use under your favourite lippy to add volume and dimension to the lips making them appear fuller with no filler.

- Highlight the bridge of your nose only if you have contoured it previously, otherwise you may end up making your nose look larger, longer and/or wider if you just highlight it. I don't understand the pixie nose trend of highlighting the tip of the nose to the extent of being able to guide Santa's sleigh.

- Once you have applied your highlighter to the areas of the face you wish to accentuate then go over these areas and buff and blend your highlighter using circular motions to create instant radiance and even tone appearance to the skin.

- Don't be afraid to wear just highlighter without any other makeup, just make sure not to overdo the glowing and end up looking greasy. In this case, I would apply highlighter just to the highest points of my face and buff them into the skin rather than applying a highlighting product over the entire face.

Baking

Okay, so I am sure you have heard the term 'baking' your makeup? But what does this actually mean to you? Baking is a technique originally used in the drag community but has been adopted by TV celebrities and some makeup artists to accompany the contouring trend. This technique is used to set foundation and concealer but the vast difference is the sheer amount of powder required to bake a makeup. You apply a lot of translucent powder on the highpoints of the face, i.e anything you would have highlighted with your lighter foundation or concealer like your chin, nose, and cheekbones. You would bake before you highlight with any illuminating products, the trick is to let the powder sit on the skin for five to ten minutes so your body heat literally bakes and sets your makeup and is supposed to leave you creaseless and flawless, however I would not recommend this technique for a mature or dry skin type.

How Do I Bake?

Once you have applied your foundation and concealer, and contoured and highlighted using a cream non-illuminating product then you are ready to bake. Grab yourself a fluffy blusher brush and sweep translucent powder over all your makeup, then wet a makeup sponge or beauty blender and pat on more translucent powder. You want to look like you have just been antiqued (smacked in the face by a bag of flour) and you are off to a good start. Let this sit for at least 10 minutes before sweeping off with that fluffy blush brush. A little trick here is to leave your makeup baking whilst you apply your eye makeup and you don't need to worry about any eyeshadow fallout as the translucent powder will capture any that may occur and it can just be swept away leaving your base flawless.

If you prefer a little bit of coverage, bit of eyeliner, lippy and off you pop, then baking is definitely not for you but for those of you who love full coverage, and a glam, strong style of makeup then give baking a try. In all my years as a makeup artist I have never 'baked' a makeup and it is not something I would do to my own face either but by all means give it a try, you may love it.

Draping

What is draping? This is the technique used to contour the face using blusher products instead of the traditional foundation or contour products that you use to define angles. Draping gives your face a softer, fresher and youthful look whilst looking more natural. I love this draping technique and it's often my go to look for the everyday when I am running errands and I just want a quick pick me up look without having to spend ages in front of the mirror with a multitude of tools, products and spending ages blending.

How Do I Drape?

You can drape your face simply using one blush product although for a look like this, I do recommend using a cream or a gel for an even application and a youthful glow. This can be applied with your fingers or using a contour brush as this is the best shape to hug those contours of the face.

Smile when applying your blush and apply to the highest points of the face for an instant lift and plumping effect on the skin.

I recommend applying your drape to your cheekbones, into the hollow start at the back near the ear and pushing the blush product back and forth to blend it out. Diffuse the blush so it melts into the skin and up the cheekbone for a natural look, ensure you don't go past the outer corner of the eye to give your face an extra lift. Draping is about lifting the contours of the face, making your cheekbones look higher and more pronounced.

If you wish to, you can use a darker blush for the hollow of the cheekbone and use a lighter blush for the cheekbone and blend it out. You could even use a bit of cream highlighter applied to the highest points of the face for extra dimension, but this may not be necessary and one colour will work just fine.

Blend your blush up towards your temples to give your face more definition and across the nose for a fun youthful look. You can also transition this into your eyeshadow too and, if you are feeling very brave, you can even apply blush to your forehead and down the nose. Pat McGrath did some extreme draping on the catwalk, creating dreamy sunsets on the models' faces incorporating the forehead, eyes and cheeks into the draped look. Now, I am not suggesting you do this but just to give you an idea of the various looks you can create with this basic technique. Your imagination is your limit, have fun with it but for an everyday look then I suggest you go for the classic draping using one colour blush.

If you have a round face, I recommend applying your drape colour slightly below the apples of the cheek as this will help lengthen your face and minimise its width.

If you apply too much blush, don't fret. You can buff over the top with a loose setting powder to mute down the tones for the perfect natural flush.

CONTOUR BRUSHES

I would recommend having a different shape brush for every step of your makeup routine, especially for contouring. You want to be using the correct shape brush suited for the job as this will make a huge difference to the appearance of your makeup finish and it may even help you speed up your application. Using a different brush for each step of your contour makeup will prevent your products and colours from becoming muddy.

Concealer Brushes

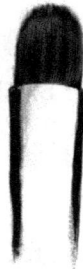

A concealer brush is used for applying cream and liquid concealer to the skin. The concealer brush looks similar to the flat eyeshadow brush but is usually slightly narrower. The dense shape makes it great for applying cream concealer. Another shape of concealer brush is the same as the crease brush and is great for blending and buffing concealer into the skin. Often cream concealers will come with their own applicator.

Contour Brushes

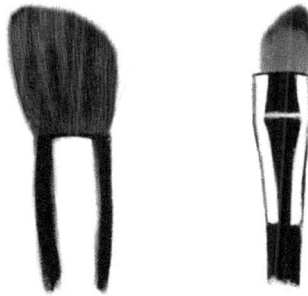

You can tell the difference between a contour brush and a blusher brush by the angled shape of the bristles. The angled shape allows for you to follow the contours of your face and easily chisel out your cheek bones and jawline. You get various sizes of contour brushes that are designed to be used on different areas of the face. The smaller brush size is used to contour your nose and eyes, it can also be used to apply contour products precisely before being blended with a larger contour brush. The softer fluffier contour brushes are great for applying blush, bronzer and highlighter whereas contour brushes with stiffer denser bristles can be used for applying contouring products. The contour brush can be used with powder, liquid and cream, just make sure it is cleaned before switching between these products to prevent them from becoming muddied.

I recommend using this brush shape for applying your blush draping as this will allow for precise application and will hug the natural contours of the face for the most natural and effective result.

Top tip – a good rule to follow when contouring the face is only use powder on top of powder and cream on cream or liquid. Apply your cream or liquid foundation, then when you are contouring using cream or liquid, apply this on top and blend it in before setting it all with translucent powder. If you are going to contour using powder then make sure you have set your foundation before applying any powder products to the skin to prevent them from sticking and being impossible to blend effectively. The same rules apply to blusher, if you are using a powder blush make sure your foundation and contour are set with powder before you apply your blush.

Blusher Brushes

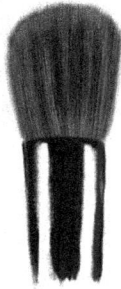

Blusher brushes are usually domed or rounded and come in a variety of different sizes. The smaller size is great for a precise application of blush to the apple of the cheek and the larger blush brush can be used to blend the blusher and buff on setting powder. The blusher brush is suitable to use with cream or powder. I tend to use a small to medium size brush for my blusher application as I find it gives a nice accurate pop of colour wherever you need it on the cheek but it also blends well into the skin. I would not recommend using a large blusher brush to apply your blush as you could end up dispersing the blusher too far across the face and distorting the shape of the face.

Powder Brush/Sponge

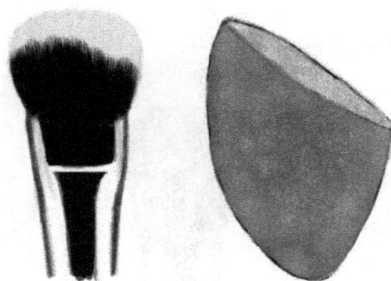

A powder brush is practically the same shape as a blusher brush but is slightly larger and has longer fluffy bristles. It is used for dusting loose or pressed powder onto the face to set makeup. This shaped brush is in literally every brush set you would ever buy and is a must have for any makeup kit.

A powder puff can be used to press on loose powder and will give you a fuller coverage.

A moist beauty blender or makeup sponge is best used to pat on your translucent powder if you want to bake your makeup.

Fan Brush

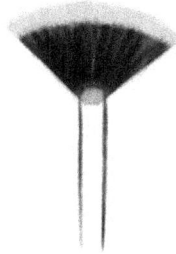

This is a brush you always get in a makeup brush set. Its soft fanned bristles makes it the perfect brush to delicately apply highlighter and bronzer and it can also be used to blend away fallout from eyeshadow or dust off excess powder.

Pointed Highlighter Brush

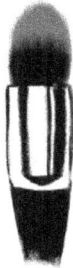

This brush looks similar to a small blusher brush but instead of getting wider towards the tip of the bristles, it gets narrower or tapered allowing for precise application of highlighter products and is suitable for powders, creams and liquids. The shape gives the brush the ability to gently buff product into the skin to create that glow or strobe lit from within look.

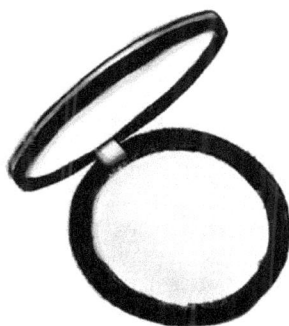

14. BLUSH

Blush gives such a great effect of waking up your face, but it can easily go wrong if you choose the wrong product to suit your skin type, the wrong tone or if you're too heavy-handed with your application.

In real life, blush should subtly complement the rest of your makeup, ideally without distraction so that it enhances whilst letting your eyes and lips do the talking.

This chapter is a guide to help you choose a blush product, shades and application tool and techniques that are going to be perfect on your skin.

TYPES

Powder Blush

I have been using powder blushers since I was little. I remember trying on my mum's makeup and ending up looking like a clown with rosy red cheeks.

Powder blushers are great for oily and combination skin types as they absorb the excess oil in the skin. They're not so great for a dry or mature skin as the powder has a matte finish that only perpetuates the dryness of the skin and extenuates fine lines, so I do not recommend this type of formula if you have a mature skin.

Powder blush, or rouge as it was once known in the renaissance, is long-lasting. These days blushers no longer contain any lead but often contain talc and titanium dioxide which can cause flashback in photographs so try to purchase a HD powder blush or check the ingredients first if you intend to wear this type of blush for an event that requires photography.

Powder blushes tend to be highly pigmented so they can sometimes look a little overpowering on a very pale skin. They are best applied with a light hand and blended well. Don't forget to set your base before applying a powder blush, otherwise your blush may cling to the base product making it difficult to blend, therefore making it difficult to achieve a natural looking result.

Cream Blush

Cream blushers are moisturising and are most suitable for dry and mature skins. The cream formula provides a beautiful, youthful natural flush to the face with a dewy finish and melts into the skin, giving a more natural finish to your makeup. Cream blushers are sheerer than powder, so they are easier to build up to the intensity you desire.

Cream blushers will set quickly so they do require a speedy application as once they are set, they are near on impossible to blend and can cause unnatural streaks on the skin if not buffed whilst damp.

Cream blushers do not stay as fresh on the skin as powder formulas do, but they will last for about 7 hours. After that you may want to think about reapplying a dab of blush.

Cream blushers can be easily applied with a finger so it is easy to reapply on the go, just make sure you wash your hands afterwards to prevent your fingers becoming stained and transferring blush onto anything else accidently, or use a beauty blender and you will be good to go.

Gel Blush

Gel blushers are suitable for all skin types. They give a beautiful sheer wash of water colour to the cheek that act like a stain without any texture, providing you with the most realistic natural result you can wish for with your blush.

Stain/Tint Blush

Like a gel formula, the stain has excellent staying power, however they require an experienced hand to apply them because they dry so fast, you have to be precise with the application and blend quickly. Stains are also not a great formula to use with a dry skin as, similar to the powder blush, the tint will cling to drier areas on the skin causing blotchy patchy makeup and no one wants that from their blush.

Cream to Powder Blush

This type of formula allows for the ease of application of a cream so you can use your fingers to apply it, but it also offers the longevity of a powder as it dries to a powder finish. This type of product is good for an oily skin type. The finish of this formula is not quite as natural as the normal cream blush but I think it makes up for it with its durability.

I wouldn't say one formula is better than another as it all depends on the look you want to achieve and your skin type. With that being said, these days cream and gels seem to have become very popular and most makeup brands will have a cream or gel version of a blush you can try.

Hopefully this will help you choose a suitable formula that you will love and that will suit you and your skin.

COLOURS

If you are anything like me, you can't go anywhere

without at least a pop of blush. I am going to help you choose a blush colour that will suit you whether you want to achieve a fresh face natural look or perhaps something a little bolder and brighter. I am going to give you all the information you will ever need to help you make an informed decision on your choice of blush colour.

So, you have decided what formula of blush you want to go for but what colour should you get? Peony, tangerine, rose or maybe berry. I am going to help you decide which colours will suit you.

Blush Shades

When choosing your blush, you need to decide whether you want your blusher to pop, e.g. contrast, or to complement your skin tone. Complementary colours will appear more natural. Adding a hint of colour to the apples of the cheek will keep you looking bright and fresh-faced all day, and using a contrasting colour will keep you looking fresh-faced but on a bolder scale.

I know I have said all along about how we work with your skin undertones but when it comes to blush

it is quite fun to do the opposite and contrast a warm
skin undertone (yellow) with a cool blush tone like a
pink, and contrast a cool undertone (pink) with a
warm blush tone like coral and peach. If you want
your blush to be more natural then choose a blush
tone with the same undertones as your skin.

When choosing your blush colour, although we
can play up the undertones, you still want the blush
tones to suit your overall skin tone of fair, medium or
dark.

Undertone	Skin Tone	Complement (natural)	Contrast (pop)
Warm skin	Light/fair	Peach, coral	Soft pinks
	Medium	Deep peach	Rich pink and mauve
	Dark	Warm browns and oranges	Fuchsia and berry
Cool skin	Light/fair	Soft pinks	Peach/coral
	Medium	Rich pinks and mauve	Deep peach/coral
	Dark	Fuchsia and light berry	Orange-tangerine

Fair Skin

The best blusher shades for fair, light skin tones are soft pinks, light corals and peaches. For those of you with cool (pink) undertones, you should wear the soft pinks for a natural complementary look and wear the peach/coral shades if you want a bolder contrasting look. If you have warm (golden) undertones go for peachy, coral shades for a complementary natural look and wear the soft pinks for that added pop of colour.

Medium Skin

For medium skin tones, you want to intensify your colours so try using richer pinks, warm mauves and deeper peach/coral. For those of you with cool undertones you should wear the rich pinks and mauve shades for a complementary look and use the deep peach/coral for your colour pop. For those of you with warm undertones, you should wear the rich pink or mauve for your pop of colour and use the deep peach shades for your natural complementary look.

Dark Skin

With dark skin, I absolutely love using deep fuchsias, oranges and warm browns. If you have cool undertones then your best bet is to wear fuchsia or light berry shades for a natural look and use orange shades, like tangerine, for your pop of colour. For those of you with warm undertones, try wearing warm browns and oranges for your natural look and use the fuchsia and berry shades for your pop of colour.

BLUSH BRUSHES

The brush you should use to apply your blush with depends on what formula of blush you have chosen and the look and finish you want to achieve with your makeup, whether that be fresh-faced and natural using complementary colours or using contrasting tones for a bolder look.

I am going to help you decide what tool is best for you to apply your choice of blusher.

Blusher Brush

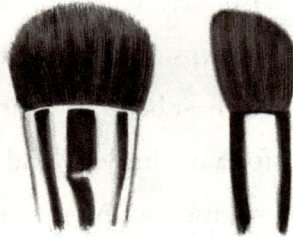

I am sure you will have all seen a blusher brush before. I think it is probably one of the most iconic brush shapes used in marketing and media.

Blusher brushes are domed or rounded and come in a variety of different sizes. The smaller size is great for a precise application of blush to the apple of the cheek and the larger blush brush can be used to blend the blusher and buff on setting powder. The blusher brush is suitable to use with cream or powder.

For sheer or medium pigmented blushers, use a big fluffy brush in a circular motion for quick effortless application. Use a smaller size of brush to apply a precise pop of colour. Make sure you blend it well with the larger blusher brush and try not to blend the blusher too far across the face otherwise you risk muddying up the face or distorting the shape of the face.

Stippling Brush

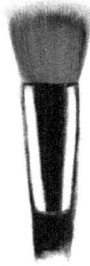

Try using a stipple brush if you want a sheerer natural finish as this type of brush picks up and deposits less colour. This is good brush to use with the stronger pigments as it allows the pigments to be applied with a light hand. This brush is suitable to use with cream and gel blushers, just dot your choice of product onto the cheek and lightly swirl to blend it in.

Beauty Blender

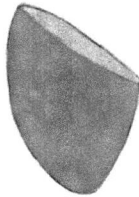

You can use a beauty blender to apply your cream or gel blush by patting and pushing the product into the skin. The blender can also be used to remove product if you have applied too much.

Fingers

Fingers are perfect for applying a cream or gel blush to the cheek. The heat from your hand helps soften and melt the product into the skin for that natural flush from within look.

15. FACE SHAPES

The seven basic face shapes are oval, round, rectangular, square, diamond, heart and oblong. Grab yourself a mirror and read on as I help you determine your face shape.

Something to think about when determining the shape of your face is it is not the overall shape that is important, it is more about the angles and contours that are essential when deciding on your face shape and this will help you decide on how you will go about contouring it.

Choosing your face shape can be a challenge if you do not know how. Often people are not just one face shape either. I have put together a few common characteristics for each face shape. I have also included four steps to accurately measure your face, to help you determine what your face shape is. Remember to take note of the angles and contours of your face to see whether they're soft, sharp, pronounced or not. Once you understand your shape, you can turn to your individual face shape section and learn how to contour, highlight, apply blusher and brow shape in a way that is perfect for your unique face.

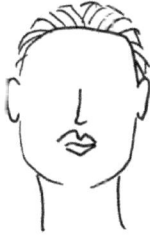

SQUARE	ROUND

Square faces are a third longer than the width of the face and have strong angles on the forehead and at the jawline.

Round faces are as wide as they are long. The cheekbones and face length are a similar measurement but tend to be larger than the forehead and jawline which are similar to one another but with soft, rounded edges.

Turn to page 276.

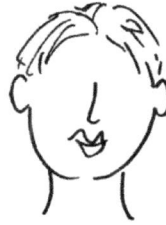

Turn to page 281.

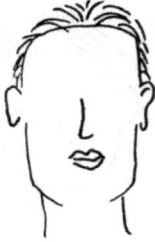

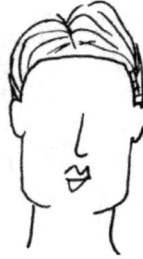

RECTANGLE

OBLONG

Rectangular faces are a third longer than the width of the face and have strong angles on the forehead and at the jawline. Elongated features from forehead to chin, some have a pronounced chin.

Oblong faces are as long as they are wide. Straight sides, a high forehead and a larger than average distance between the bottom of the lip and the tip of the chin are common attributes of the oblong face.

Turn to page 288.

Turn to page 293.

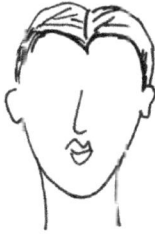

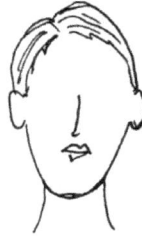

HEART	OVAL

Heart-shaped faces have the most width at the cheek, eye and forehead areas, with a narrow to pointy chin. Sometimes they will also have a high prominent forehead or a widows peak (a V-shaped point in the hairline at the centre of the forehead).

Oval-shaped faces have an overall length larger than the width of the cheekbones, and the forehead and jaw are equal widths. With prominent cheekbones, the face gradually tapers towards the chin.

Turn to page 298.

Turn to page 304.

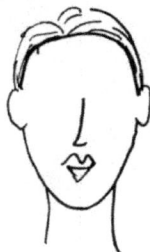

DIAMOND

Diamond-shaped faces are characterised by a narrow forehead and a narrow chin with the widest point at the cheeks. The length is often the largest measurement or is the same as the width. This is a less common face shape.

Turn to page 310.

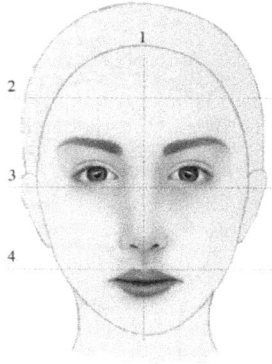

Measuring Your Face

This is how to actually measure your face to find your face shape:

1) Forehead: measure the distance across your forehead at the widest point, from hairline to hairline.

2) Cheekbones: measure across your upper cheeks, starting and ending at the sharp bump below the outer corner of each eye.

3) Jawline: measure your jaw across your face at its widest point (about an inch down from your ears).

4) Face length: measure from the centre of your hairline to the tip of your chin.

SQUARE FACE SHAPE

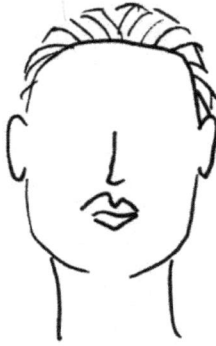

If you have a square-shaped face, your temples, cheekbones and jawline have defined angles and you most likely have a straight hairline. Your face is the same length as width and your forehead is the same width as your jaw.

Celebrities with your face shape include Demi Lovato and Katie Holmes.

I am going to give you all the know-how to help you complement, balance and flatter your unique face shape with subtle contouring, a complementary blush and a balanced brow.

How To Contour and Highlight Your Face Shape

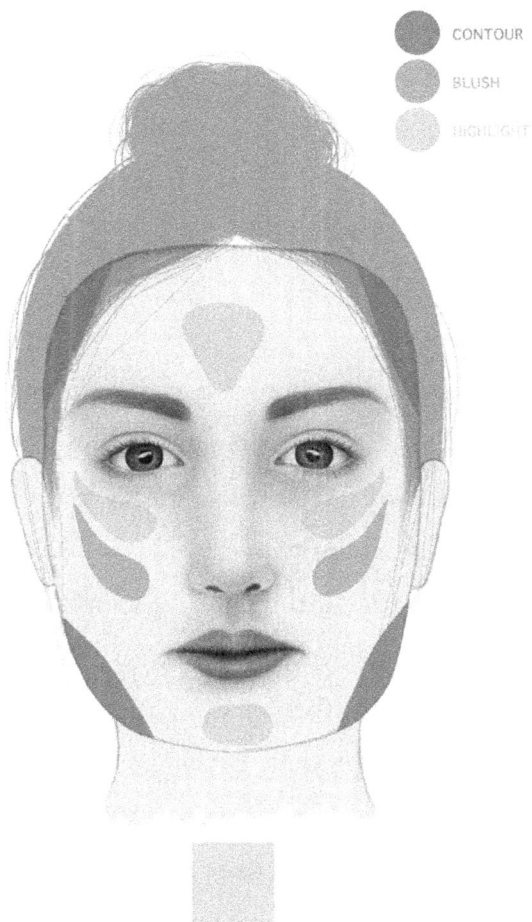

The most important thing you need to remember when contouring your face is that highlighting brings a feature forward while accentuating and enlarging,

whereas applying a darker shade will push the features back and make things look smaller.

When contouring a square face, the goal is to soften defined edges and round out your angular features. You'll want to contour around the perimeter of your face to soften those corners on the temples and jawline beneath the ears, and blend well to get a natural look.

Highlight does not have to mean shimmer or glow. It can also refer to creating dimension in the face by using a lighter coloured base product as I talked about in the Contouring chapter of this book. This process enhances facial features and draws more attention to that area of the face.

To make the face appear longer with your choice of highlighter product, apply highlight to the centre of your forehead, chin and tops of the cheekbones.

I recommend using a fan brush for applying any glittery, shimmery powder products, and a pointed highlighter brush or a small contour brush for applying any creamy products.

Where To Apply Your Blusher

You should have already decided on your choice of blush formula and colour, and chosen whether you want your blush to complement and look natural or if you want your blush to pop and contrast for a bolder look. This can be applied with a light hand so you can still achieve something deemed natural but in a bolder palette.

Refer to the chapter on blusher to choose your suitable blush formula, colour and tool for application.

Remember, if you want your blush to pop on the skin then you want to choose the opposite undertone to your skin tone. If you want your blush to be natural then choose the blush undertone in a cool or warm to match your skin's natural undertone.

Apply your choice of blush under the apples of the cheek (the plumpest part of the cheek) under the cheekbone, directly in line with the pupil, and blend upwards towards the tops of the ears to create a tear drop shape for the most flattering blush for a square face.

How To Define and Shape Your Brow To Complement Your Square Face

Choosing flattering brows is all about selecting a brow shape that will complement and balance out your unique face shape.

High curved, rounded arches will help soften angles across the forehead and jawline, which will make a square face appear longer and narrower with softer angles. Make sure you don't extend the brow tail too far down the face as this will likely make your eyes appear downturned.

I recommend using an angled brush to apply your cream, liquid, gels, powders or pomade brow products for a precise controlled application.

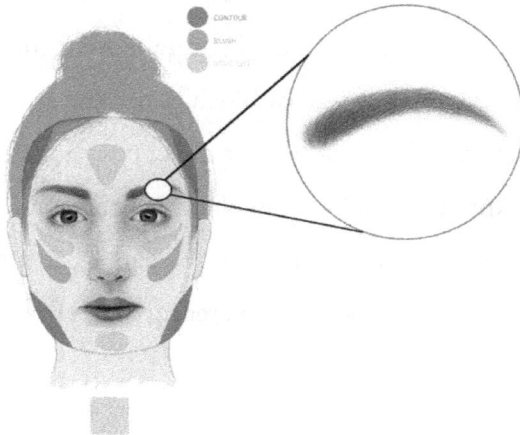

ROUND FACE SHAPE

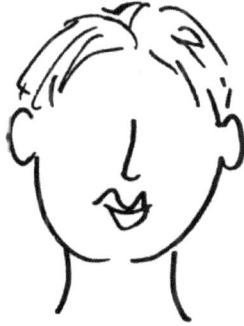

Round faces are as wide as they are long, the cheekbones tend to be the widest part with softer angles and edges, and the jawline is rounded. A round face does not mean you have a big face, you can have a petite round face.

Celebrities with your face shape include Gabrielle Union, Ginnifer Goodwin, Mila Kunis and Kirsten Dunst.

I am going to give you all the know-how to help you complement, balance and flatter your unique face shape with subtle contouring, a complementary blush and a balanced brow.

How To Contour and Highlight Your Face Shape

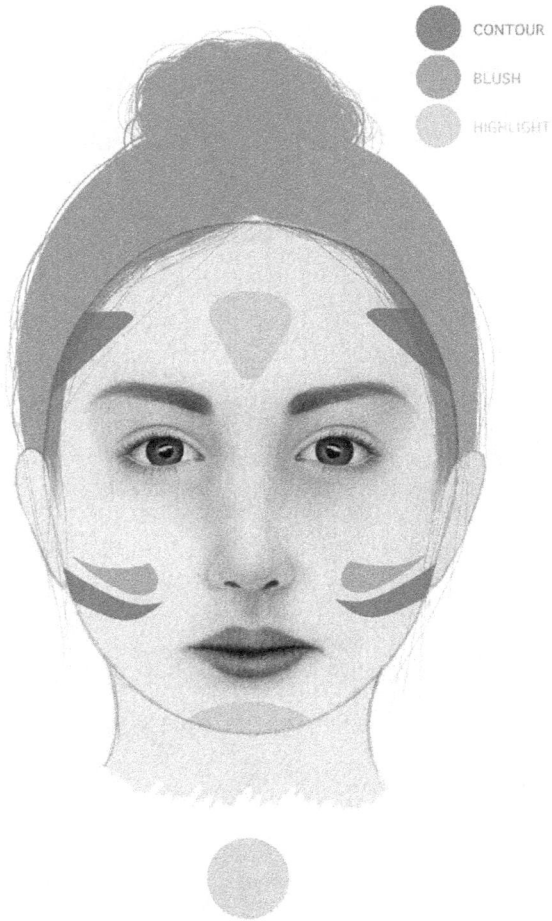

CONTOUR

BLUSH

HIGHLIGHT

Once you have applied your base, the definition can often be lost on a round face so the key to contouring a round face is to create shadows, definition and create the effect of angles.

The most important thing you need to remember when contouring your face is that highlighting brings a feature forward while accentuating and enlarging, whereas applying a darker shade will push the features back and make things look smaller.

Using your choice of contour product, either cream or powder based, you want to shade the perimeter of the face along the edge of the hair, near the temples. You do not want to contour across the entire forehead, apply contour only to the jawline and under the cheekbones. If you follow where the top of the ear connects to the side of the head and follow the cheekbone down into the centre of the face, making sure you do not shade past where the natural outer edge of the eye sits, this will give your face a natural lift. Don't be afraid to have a feel of your face, you want the shade to sit in the hollows of the cheek bones but with that being said, you are still trying to lift the cheekbone so you don't want to shade too far down the face. You want the product to sit slightly on the cheekbone to really give a lift to the face. I recommend using a contour brush as this shape brush

really helps hug the natural contours of the face and if
you use a small contour brush you can map out your
contouring and then use a softer, fluffier contour
brush to blend it all together. The most important
step of contouring is blending. You are trying to
create the effect of natural shadows in the skin, a
harsh unblended line will be a dead giveaway. Be sure
to start subtly and apply makeup in natural light to get
the best results.

When contouring your jawline, a great tip to try is
to apply the product right on the edge of the jawline.
If you go too far underneath the jaw you can actually
end up making a round face look rounder and larger,
this is also a good technique to use if you have a
double chin.

Highlight does not have to mean shimmer or glow.
It can also refer to creating dimension in the face
using a lighter coloured base product, as I mentioned
in the Contouring chapter of this book. This process
enhances those features and draws more attention to
that area of the face.

With a round face shape you want to apply

highlight across the highest point on your cheekbones and between your contour line and jaw, i.e. contour under the cheekbone and then apply your highlight directly beneath, this will create some realistic angles resulting in a more sculptured look.

I recommend using a fan brush for applying any glittery, shimmery powder products, and a pointed highlighter brush or a small contour brush for applying any creamy products.

Where To Apply Your Blusher

You should have already decided on your choice of blush formula and colour, and chosen whether you want your blush to complement and look natural or if you want your blush to pop and contrast for a bolder look. This can be applied with a light hand so you can still achieve something deemed natural but in a bolder palette.

Refer to the chapter on blusher to choose your suitable blush formula, colour and tool for application.

Remember, if you want your blush to pop on the skin then you want to choose the opposite undertone to your skin tone. If you want your blush to be natural then choose the blush undertone in a cool or warm to match your skin's natural undertone.

Apply your choice of blush under the apples of the cheek (the plumpest part of the cheek) nearest the nose and blend upwards towards the top of the ears to create definition on a round face shape.

How To Define and Shape Your Brow To Complement Your Round Face

Choosing flattering eyebrows is all about selecting a brow shape that will complement and balance out your unique face shape.

I recommend using an angled brush to apply your cream, liquid, gels, powders or pomade brow products for a precise controlled application.

A fuller, lifted arched brow on a round face will add length, definition, and sharpness to an otherwise soft-angled face.

Be careful not to extend your arch further out than the outer edge of the iris as this could make your face appear wider than it is.

If you have a small round face, try not to

overwhelm your face with brows that are too thick
and fluffy.

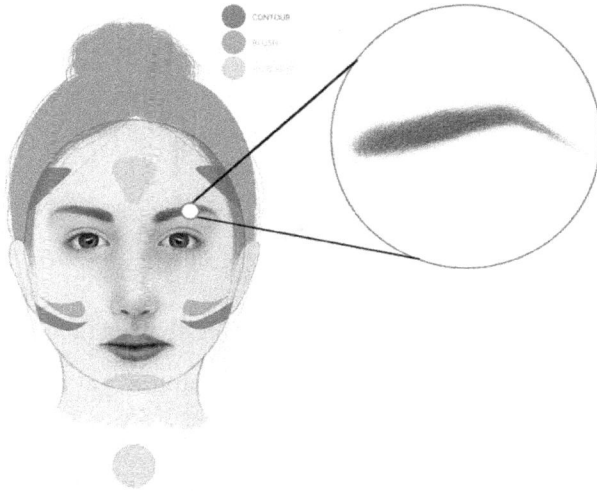

RECTANGLE FACE SHAPE

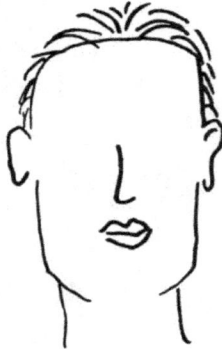

You have a rectangle-shaped face if your face is longer than its width with strong angles on the forehead and at the jawline. You most likely have a particularly straight hairline and elongated features, such as the forehead and chin, and you may have a pronounced chin.

Celebrities with your face shape include Kate Winslet and Angelina Jolie.

I am going to give you all the know-how to help you complement, balance and flatter your unique face shape with subtle contouring, a complementary blush and a balanced brow.

How To Contour and Highlight Your Face Shape

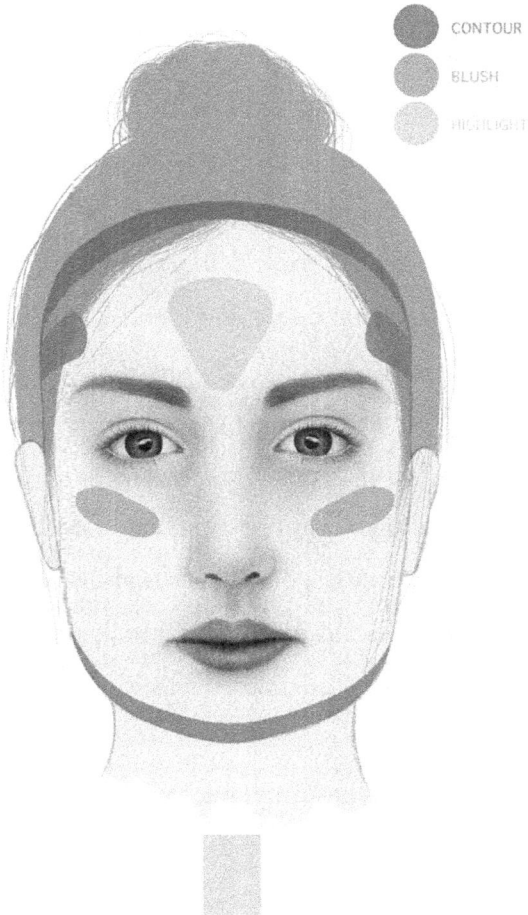

CONTOUR

BLUSH

HIGHLIGHT

The most important thing you need to remember
when contouring your face is that highlighting brings
a feature forward while accentuating and enlarging,

whereas applying a darker shade will push the features back and make things look smaller.

When contouring a rectangle face, the goal is to soften defined edges and round out your angular features. You'll want to contour around the perimeter of your forehead along the hairline, temples and along the entire jawline to help shorten the appearance of the face and make sure you blend it well to get a natural look.

I recommend using a contour brush for applying your choice of contour product. If you don't feel as confident in your application, use a small contour brush to map out your shadows and then buff into the skin using a fluffier larger brush and build it up slowly until you are happy with it.

Highlight does not have to mean shimmer or glow. It can also refer to creating dimension in the face using a lighter coloured base product, as I mentioned in the Contouring chapter of this book. This process enhances those features and draws more attention to that area of the face.

When it comes to a highlighting a rectangle face shape you don't need to use much, just a little bit applied to the centre of the forehead is all you will need.

I recommend using a fan brush for applying any glittery, shimmery powder products, and a pointed highlighter brush or a small contour brush for applying any creamy products.

Where To Apply Your Blusher

You should have already decided on your choice of blush formula and colour, and chosen whether you want your blush to complement and look natural or if you want your blush to pop and contrast for a bolder look. This can be applied with a light hand so you can still achieve something deemed natural but in a bolder palette.

Refer to the chapter on blusher to choose your suitable blush formula, colour and tool for application.

Remember, if you want your blush to pop on the skin then you want to choose the opposite undertone to your skin tone. If you want your blush to be natural then choose the blush undertone in a cool or warm to match your skin's natural undertone.

Apply your choice of blush under the apples of the cheek (the plumpest part of the cheek) directly in line with the pupil and blend outwards for the most flattering blush for your face.

How To Define and Shape Your Brow To Complement Your Rectangle Face

A straighter shorter brow with a straight arch will make a long face appear fuller and shorter.

I recommend using an angled brush to apply your cream, liquid, gels, powders or pomade brow products for a precise controlled application.

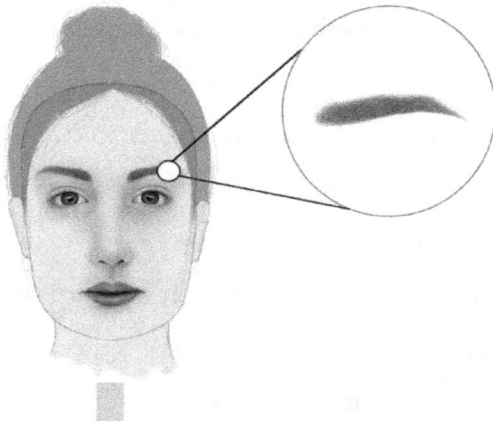

OBLONG FACE SHAPE

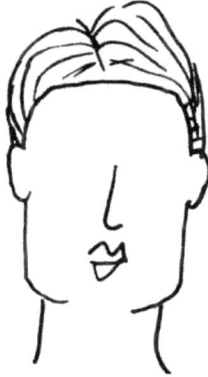

Oblong faces are as long as they are wide. Common attributes of the oblong face are relatively straight sides, lacking cheekbone definition, with a high forehead and a larger than average distance between the bottom of the lip and the tip of the chin.

Celebrities with a diamond face shape include Sarah Jessica Parker and Liv Tyler.

I am going to give you all the know-how to help you complement, balance and flatter your unique face shape with subtle contouring, a complementary blush and a balanced brow.

How To Contour and Highlight Your Face Shape

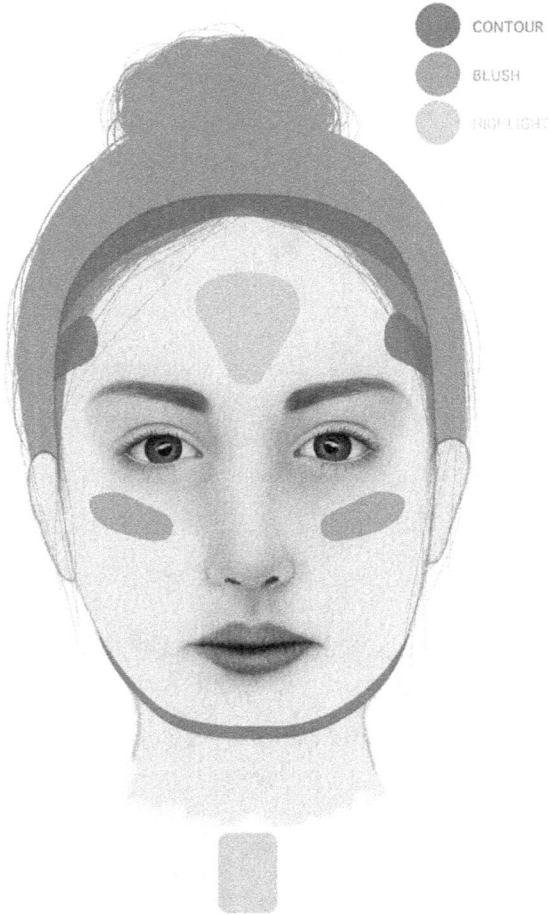

The most important thing you need to remember when contouring your face is that highlighting brings a feature forward while accentuating and enlarging,

whereas applying a darker shade will push the features back and make things look smaller.

Using your choice of contour product, either cream or powder based, you want to shade the perimeter of the forehead along the hairline and into the temples to soften and minimise the width of the forehead. Apply a little contour along the jawline, from edge to edge, to shorten the length of the face and add definition to the jaw.

I recommend using a contour brush as this shape brush really helps hug the natural contours of the face and if you use a small contour brush you can map out your contouring and then use a softer fluffier contour brush to blend it all together. The most important step of contouring is blending, you are trying to create the effect of natural shadows in the skin, a harsh unblended line will be a dead giveaway. Be sure to start subtly and apply makeup in natural light to get the best results.

Highlight does not have to mean shimmer or glow. It can also refer to creating dimension in the face using a lighter coloured base product, as I mentioned

Make Up Your Face

in the Contouring chapter of this book. This process enhances those features and draws more attention to that area of the face.

With a heart shape face, you want to use very little highlighter, if any, applied to the centre of the forehead.

Where To Apply Your Blusher

You should have already decided on your choice of blush formula and colour, and chosen whether you want your blush to complement and look natural or if you want your blush to pop and contrast for a bolder look. This can be applied with a light hand so you can still achieve something deemed natural but in a bolder palette.

Refer to the chapter on blusher to choose your suitable blush formula, colour and tool for application.

Remember, if you want your blush to pop on the skin then you want to choose the opposite undertone to your skin tone. If you want your blush to be natural then choose the blush undertone in a cool or warm to match your skin's natural undertone.

Apply your choice of blusher to the very top of the apples of the cheek, keeping the placement central and no wider than the natural eye length.

How To Define and Shape Your Brow To Complement Your Oblong Shaped Face

Choosing flattering eyebrows is all about selecting a brow shape that will complement and balance out your unique face shape.

I recommend using an angled brush to apply your cream, liquid, gels, powders or pomade brow products for a precise controlled application.

A shorter, straighter brow with soft edges can help widen the face shape or even a fluffier thicker brow can be carried well on this face shape and will help shorten its length.

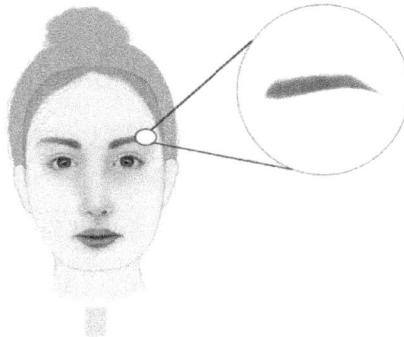

HEART FACE SHAPE

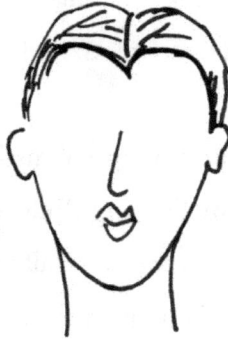

Heart-shaped faces have the most width at the cheek, eye and forehead areas, with a narrow to pointy chin and this face shape is often longer than it is wide. They may have a high prominent forehead with a rounded hairline or even a widow's peak (a V-shaped point in the hairline at the center of the forehead).

Celebrities with the heart-shaped face include Halle Berry, Reese Witherspoon and Jennifer Love Hewitt.

I am going to give you all the know-how to help you complement, balance and flatter your unique face shape with subtle contouring, a complementary blush and a balanced brow.

How To Contour and Highlight Your Face Shape

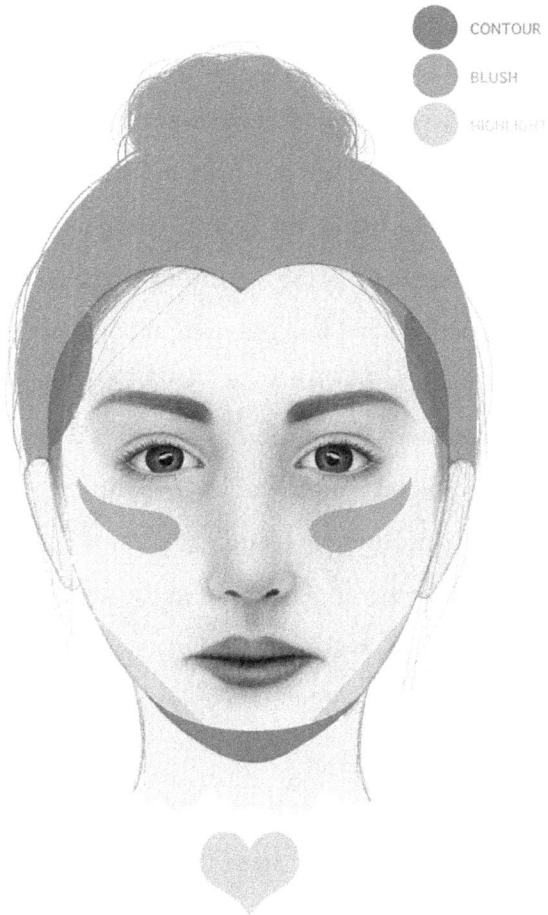

The most important thing you need to remember when contouring your face is that highlighting brings a feature forward while accentuating and enlarging,

whereas applying a darker shade will push the features back and make things look smaller.

Using your choice of contour product, either cream or powder based, you want to shade the temples to soften and minimise the width of the forehead. As you already have a defined jaw, apply a little contour below the chin to minimise its length.

I recommend using a contour brush as this shape brush really helps hug the natural contours of the face and if you use a small contour brush you can map out your contouring and then use a softer fluffier contour brush to blend it all together. The most important step of contouring is blending, you are trying to create the effect of natural shadows in the skin, a harsh unblended line will be a dead giveaway. Be sure to start subtly and apply makeup in natural light to get the best results.

Highlight does not have to mean shimmer or glow. It can also refer to creating dimension in the face using a lighter coloured base product, as I mentioned in the Contouring chapter of this book. This process enhances those features and draws more attention to that area of the face.

With a heart shape face you want to use highlight sparingly and apply it to the centre of the forehead, under the brow. If you are using an iridescent, light reflective highlighter then do not do this on a mature skin as this will make the brow appear heavier rather than lifting. Apply your highlighter to the bridge of the nose, cupid's bow and cheekbones, making sure not to go too close to the eyes as this may make the under-eye area appear puffy. Highlight the centre of the chin under the lower lip and along the edges of the jawline to help broaden that point.

Where To Apply Your Blusher

You should have already decided on your choice of blush formula and colour, and chosen whether you want your blush to complement and look natural or if you want your blush to pop and contrast for a bolder look This can be applied with a light hand so you can still achieve something deemed natural but in a bolder palette.

Refer to the chapter on blusher to choose your suitable blush formula, colour and tool for application.

Remember, if you want your blush to pop on the skin then you want to choose the opposite undertone to your skin tone. If you want your blush to be natural then choose the blush undertone in a cool or warm to match your skin's natural undertone.

Apply your choice of blusher to the top of the cheekbones starting from the middle and blending out and upwards towards the tails of the brow to help lift the face. Make sure you have set your foundation with translucent powder before applying your blush if you are choosing to use a powder blush.

How To Define and Shape Your Brow To Complement Your Heart-Shaped Face

Choosing flattering eyebrows is all about selecting a brow shape that will complement and balance out your unique face shape.

I recommend using an angled brush to apply your cream, liquid, gels, powders or pomade brow products for a precise controlled application.

A soft-rounded arch on a heart-shaped face will balance out a longer chin and soften sharper features.

Choose a thicker and fuller shaped brow, heart-shaped faces look great with a fluffier brow as this is widest part of the face and it won't look overwhelming.

If you don't have naturally fluffy brows try brushing through a pomade or cream-based brow product to help replicate hair growth and give the illusion of a thicker brow.

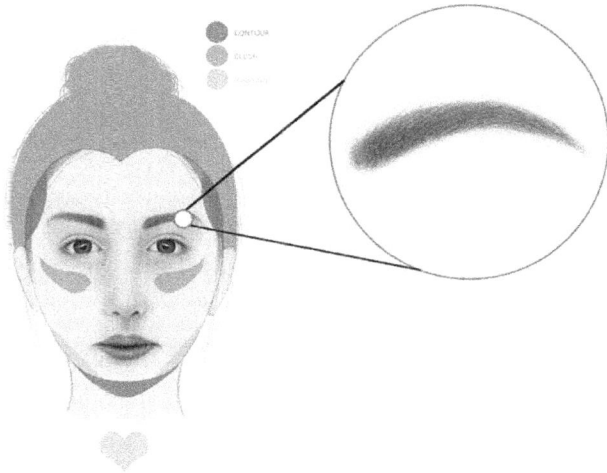

OVAL FACE SHAPE

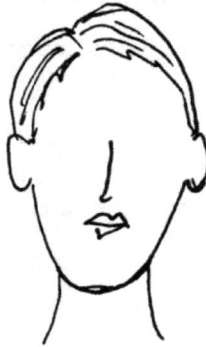

Oval-shaped faces have an overall length that is larger than the width of the cheekbones and the forehead and jaw are equal widths. An oval face features prominent cheekbones and the face gradually tapers towards the chin.

Celebrities with a diamond face shape include Jessica Alba, Beyonce and Eva Mendes.

I am going to give you all the know-how to help you complement, balance and flatter your unique face shape with subtle contouring, a complementary blush and a balanced brow.

How To Contour and Highlight Your Face Shape

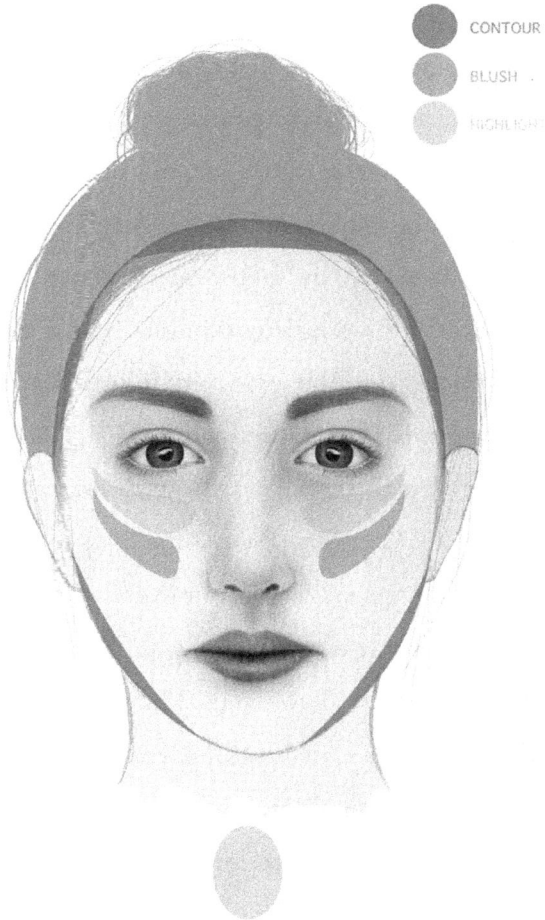

The most important thing you need to remember when contouring your face is that highlighting brings a feature forward while accentuating and enlarging,

whereas applying a darker shade will push the features back and make things look smaller.

Since your face is already symmetrical, you only need to apply a little bit of contouring, if any. Using your choice of contour product, either cream or powder based, you want to lightly shade the perimeter of the forehead along the hairline and into the temples to soften and minimise the width of the forehead. Apply a little contour along the jawline edge from underneath the earlobe to the centre of the chin, blending well for a natural shadow.

I recommend using a contour brush as this shape brush really helps hug the natural contours of the face and if you use a small contour brush you can map out your contouring and then use a softer fluffier contour brush to blend it all together. The most important step of contouring is blending, you are trying to create the effect of natural shadows in the skin, a harsh unblended line will be a dead giveaway. Be sure to start subtly and apply makeup in natural light to get the best results.

Highlight does not have to mean shimmer or glow.

It can also refer to creating dimension in the face using a lighter coloured base product, as I talked about in the Contouring chapter of this book. This process enhances those features and draws more attention to that area of the face.

With an oval shape face you want to use very little highlighter, if any, applied to the cheekbones.

Where To Apply Your Blusher

You should have already decided on your choice of blush formula and colour, and chosen whether you want your blush to complement and look natural or if you want your blush to pop and contrast for a bolder look. This can be applied with a light hand so you can still achieve something deemed natural but in a bolder palette.

Refer to the chapter on blusher to choose your suitable blush formula, colour and tool for application.

Remember, if you want your blush to pop on the skin then you want to choose the opposite undertone to your skin tone. If you want your blush to be natural then choose the blush undertone in a cool or warm to match your skin's natural undertone.

Apply your choice of blusher to the underneath of your cheekbones or the fleshiest part of the cheek to add depth and make the face look fuller, making sure you blend it up and out towards your hairline.

How To Define and Shape Your Brow To Complement Your Oval Face

Choosing flattering eyebrows is all about selecting a brow shape that will complement and balance out your unique face shape.

I recommend using an angled brush to apply your cream, liquid, gels, powders or pomade brow products for a precise controlled application.

With an oval face, I recommend that you work with your natural brow shape. Just make sure you fill in any gaps and that the brow is well measured and starts in line with the edge of your nostril and the tail ends in line with the outer corner of the eye. See the Brows chapter for information on how to measure your brow.

Make Up Your Face

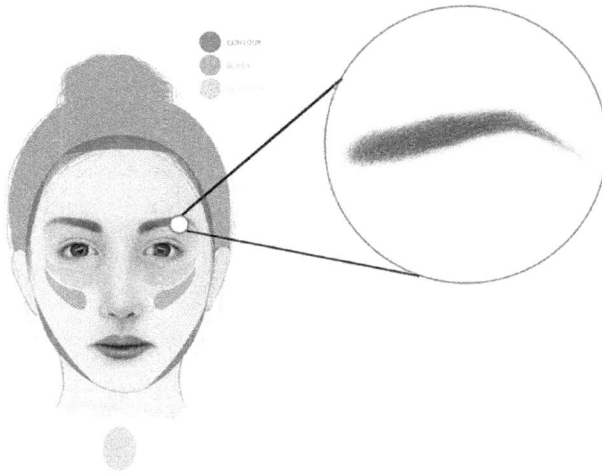

DIAMOND FACE SHAPE

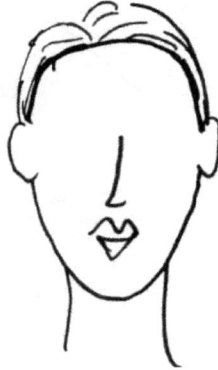

Diamond-shaped faces are characterised by a narrow forehead and a rounded narrow chin with the widest point across the cheeks, with prominent cheekbones. The length is often the largest measurement or is the same as the width.

Celebrities with a diamond face shape include Jennifer Lopez and Elizabeth Hurley.

I am going to give you all the know-how to help you complement, balance and flatter your unique face shape with subtle contouring, a complementary blush and a balanced brow.

How To Contour and Highlight Your Face Shape

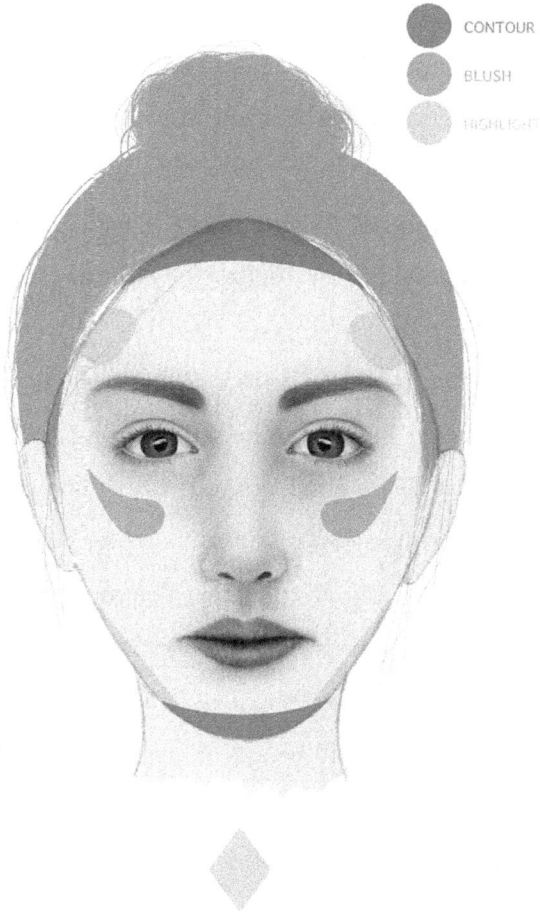

The most important thing you need to remember when contouring your face is that highlighting brings a feature forward while accentuating and enlarging,

whereas applying a darker shade will push the features back and make things look smaller.

Using your choice of contour product, either cream or powder based, you want to shade the perimeter of the face across the top of forehead, along the hairline, to soften and minimise the width of the forehead. As you already have a defined jaw, apply a little contour below the chin to minimise its length.

I recommend using a contour brush as this shape brush really helps hug the natural contours of the face and if you use a small contour brush you can map out your contouring and then use a softer fluffier contour brush to blend it all together. The most important step of contouring is blending, you are trying to create the effect of natural shadows in the skin, a harsh unblended line will be a dead giveaway. Be sure to start subtly and apply makeup in natural light to get the best results.

Highlight does not have to mean shimmer or glow. It can also refer to creating dimension in the face using a lighter coloured base product, as I mentioned in the Contouring chapter of this book. This process enhances those features and draws more attention to that area of the face.

With a diamond shape face you want to use highlighter sparingly applied to the temples and jawline to help maximise and make these areas appear broader.

Where To Apply Your Blusher

You should have already decided on your choice of blush formula and colour, and chosen whether you want your blush to complement and look natural or if you want your blush to pop and contrast for a bolder look. This can be applied with a light hand so you can still achieve something deemed natural but in a bolder palette.

Refer to the chapter on blusher to choose your suitable blush formula, colour and tool for application.

Remember, if you want your blush to pop on the skin then you want to choose the opposite undertone to your skin tone. If you want your blush to be natural then choose the blush undertone in a cool or warm to match your skin's natural undertone.

Apply your choice of blusher to the top of the cheekbones, starting from the middle and blending out and upwards towards the tails of the brow to help lift the face. Make sure you have set your foundation with translucent powder before applying your blush if you are choosing to use a powder blush.

How To Define and Shape Your Brow To Complement Your Heart-Shaped Face

Choosing flattering eyebrows is all about selecting a brow shape that will complement and balance out your unique face shape.

I recommend using an angled brush to apply your cream, liquid, gels, powders or pomade brow products for a precise controlled application.

A curved brow with an angled arch will help lengthen the widest part of the face.

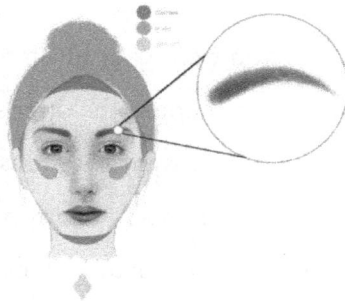

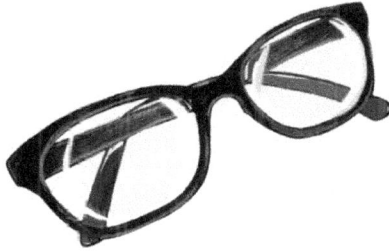

16. MAKEUP FOR THOSE WHO WEAR GLASSES

Here are some everyday techniques for applying your makeup to wear with your glasses.

Glasses can change your entire look. You can choose to complement your glasses and make your eyes stand out or dress up your lips for drama.

I have created this section just for you, for when you wear glasses. I have given lots of hints and techniques to help wake up your makeup underneath your glasses.

First of all, I know it can be a struggle to apply makeup when you wear glasses as you are unable to clearly see what you are doing without wearing them.

I recommend investing in a magnifying light up mirror, you can get some that attach directly on to your ordinary mirror. Always make sure you are applying your makeup in as much natural daylight as possible in a well-lit room to begin with. Try using makeup brushes that have a shorter handle to give you even better control for a precise application and use your little finger where possible to rest on your face to give you more stability when applying your details.

Brows

Although your glasses frame your eyes, your brows need to frame your glasses so make sure you groom your brows and fill in any sparse areas or gaps with your choice of brow pomade, gel, powder or pencil. Make sure you tidy up the edges and pluck any stray hairs to keep your brows looking neat and groomed as they will be magnified behind your lenses.

To complement a thin frame on your glasses, I recommend keeping your brows thinner and vice versa, if you have a thicker frame then go for a thicker brow with a strong arch. You don't want the brow to be the focal point of the face but you do want to complement your face and most importantly your glasses.

Lashes

For daytime, I suggest you keep your lashes soft and fluffy. Glasses can magnify your lashes so make sure you remove any lumps from your mascara by combing through the lashes after applying your favorite mascara. I recommend using a waterproof mascara that boosts volume rather than length and curl your lashes to open up your eyes and ensure that the lashes do not touch the lenses.

If you are feeling daring, why not try applying a coloured mascara over the top of a black, applied towards the tip to give your lashes a nice tint without being too overdramatic.

If you choose to apply false lashes then I recommend using lashes that emphasis volume rather than length as lengthy lashes will likely rub on your lenses and become irritating throughout the day.

Eyeliner

Some glasses can make eyes appear smaller. In order to counteract this effect use a nude eyeliner applied to your lower waterline and inner corner to help open up the eye and make it appear larger. You can also use a pop of highlighter in the inner corner of the eye to help open up and awaken the eye further.

If your lenses magnify the eye, try lining your entire eye including the waterline to make it appear smaller.

I suggest matching your eyeliner thickness to your glasses frame. If your frames are thicker, you want to apply a thicker line to the upper lash line to make your eyes stand out. If you want a flick then aim it at the top corner of your frame, this will elongate the eye and make it appear larger.

If your frames are thinner, then a softer thin line across your upper lash line works really well. It's important to make sure that there is balance between the definition of your frames and your eyes to help your eyes stand out.

Don't be afraid to play with coloured eyeliner too. Try using a coloured kohl or gel instead of your normal brown or black liner, you could choose to match the colour to your frames for a truly unique look.

Eyeshadows

A neutral palette works best behind glasses. This is not to say that it has to be boring and lack colour, you can still use colours and shimmery shades too.

Using a shadow that is lighter and brighter than your frames will help make your eyes stand out. If you want to work in the same colour as your frame, make sure you go a shade lighter on the lid and a shade darker in the crease to give the eye more shape and definition. You don't want the colour of your eyeshadow to compete with your glasses, you want it to complement them.

I recommend applying a matte warm tone to the crease and slightly above the crease with a soft crease brush and blend well. Apply a lighter tone like a beige or cream shadow, this can be matte or shimmer, to the eyelid with a flat shader brush to make the eyes appear larger.

Always finish with eyeliner and mascara.

Concealer

If you wear thicker, darker frames then these can often cast shadows under the eyes. This can prove to be quite problematic for people who also have natural dark circles under their eyes, as the lenses often magnifies any discolouration or darkness.

You can counteract this by blending a peach-toned concealer beneath the lower eyelids to correct the darkness and use a skin-toned concealer over the top. Make sure you set this area with translucent powder to prevent any product transferring onto your glasses. The eye area tends to get a little sweatier when you wear glasses, you can combat this by applying a setting spray over the top of your eye makeup. I also recommend using a setting powder applied with a pointed highlighter brush or crease brush so you can precisely set the undereye area.

Try using an eyeshadow primer instead of your normal face primer on the bridge of the nose where your nose pads of your glasses sit to help prevent your glasses from slipping and wearing off your makeup through the day.

Foundation

There is no special foundation available for glass wearers but there are a few simple steps you can take to prolong your foundation and prevent it from slipping and transferring to your frames.

Apply your foundation like normal with your choice of brush or sponge, I would suggest applying it after your eye makeup but before concealer as you will find you won't need to use as much concealer this way.

Apply your foundation all over the face but before you set your makeup, use a dampened beauty blender to blot off any excess product on the bridge of the nose, tops of the cheeks, and anywhere where your glasses naturally sit. Roll the sponge in a dabbing action to lift off the excess product to prevent unwanted transfer, then dust the setting powder on these areas to stop your glasses from sticking to your foundation and removing it.

You don't have to set the entire face if you don't want to, you can spot set the problem areas like the bridge of the nose, under the eye and cheeks, and apply a setting spray over the rest of the face.

Lips

Have you thought about ditching the eye makeup all together and just concentrating on making your lips the focal point of your makeup? Why not try a pink, red, a more exotic mauve lip or a burgundy lip. This suits most skin tones and hair colours. A bright bold lip with glasses will really brighten up the face. Choose pretty shades of pink for your lips and cheeks to give contrast to a darker, thicker frame.

Make sure you moisturise and exfoliate those lips before trying this look and don't forget to groom your brows for a more polished put together look.

If you want to do an eye makeup and a bold lip, of course you can. A bold lip with classic eyes would look fantastic. I suggest working with your glasses's undertone, for example if your frames are warmer toned then use warm-toned eyeshadow and lipstick for a harmonious complementary look.

I hope you find these tips helpful for creating your everyday makeup looks to suit you and your frames, and remember these are only guidelines and whatever you feel the most beautiful in is only going to make you more confident.

Glasses are a fashion statement, just like your clothes and makeup, so have fun playing with each element and experiment to find the right look for you.

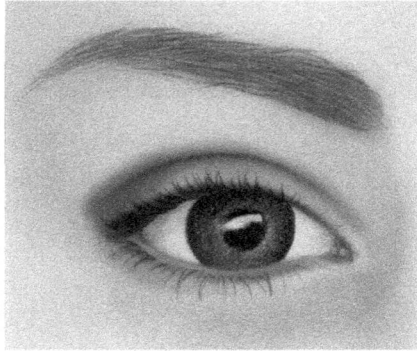

17. NATURAL MAKEUP

The most common request that I get from my brides and clients is a "natural makeup" look but what does that actually mean? I know that your version of natural would be different to mine. You can create a range of looks from barely there, the no makeup look, to soft glam and it can still be considered "natural".

In this section, when discussing natural makeup we are going to be focusing on the skin, eyes and lips and using products to enhance your features instead of disguising flaws to create a natural look to see you through all occasions from school and work to date nights whilst remaining natural.

Natural makeup takes a minimalist approach using

less product therefore it is a faster simpler application. Natural makeup will look totally different on everyone, which is something I love about this style.

The best natural looking makeup will highlight your best assets, whether that's flawless skin, pretty eyes or voluptuous lips. It will enhance your features rather than disguise flaws. You don't need to know any complex application techniques or use specific tools as your fingers will work just fine for this type of look.

I have created a step-by-step guide that uses less than ten products for the entire face, including skincare, and developed a short guide for creating a soft natural smoky eye.

Skin

With any makeup application, the key to a great look is a clean canvas to work on. This is even more important when it comes to creating a natural look as you will be using less product on the skin and using sheerer products so your skin shines through, so you want your skin to be in the best condition that it can be before attempting a natural look.

I am not pretending that I am a dermatologist and know absolutely everything about the skin because I don't; but I do know that looking after your skin with a good skincare routine, removing all your makeup before sleeping and moisturising before applying makeup is a must.

When looking after your skin or prepping your skin for a natural makeup look, it's essential to tackle any skin issues such as dry areas and acne. Use a cleanser to remove dirt and oil from the skin, toner to even out skin tone and moisturise before applying an SPF and your choice of primer. I highly recommend applying primer before any makeup application as this will prolong your makeup by giving it something to adhere to, blur imperfections, pores and fine lines and give you a smooth base to work on.

I recommend using a type of moisturiser that suits your skin type but if all else fails then use a light moisturiser without perfume to prevent skin irritation.

Don't be afraid to use different types of primer for different areas of the face, for example, if you suffer from enlarged pores then use a poreless primer on those problem areas. If you don't have a primer then spray a setting spray onto your skin and apply a thin layer of translucent powder to create a clean canvas to work on.

If you want to speed up this part of the process then use a BB cream as this product combines moisturiser, primer and SPF all together for a speedy application. This can, in fact, be used instead of foundation for a barely there look.

Foundation

When creating a natural makeup look you want to use a foundation that provides a light to medium coverage as a fuller coverage will likely look too thick on the skin and erase your features. You want your skin to shine through. I suggest using a liquid formula that suits your skin type and tones for the best results. Choose a formula with a dewy or satin finish for the most natural looking finish. You could add a hint of liquid illuminator to your foundation for an even more fresh, dewy glow.

The application is the most critical step to creating your natural looking foundation. Whatever your choice of tool, whether it's a damp sponge, brush or your fingers, make sure that you apply it sparingly. You may not need to apply it all over the face, you can just apply it where you require a little correction and coverage. Blend around your hairline and down onto your neck to prevent any unseemly tide lines.

Concealer

As with foundation, you want to use your concealer sparingly and precisely on any problem areas such as dark circles, imperfections and acne. Select a formula that matches your foundation so that it blends seamlessly. Use two different shades of concealer, one which is the same shade as your foundation for using on blemishes and another one to two shades lighter for a brightening effect to use under the eyes. Apply your concealer with a soft fluffy brush and use your finger to pat the concealer in and blend it into the skin. Set with a dusting of setting powder.

Blush

Blush can really brighten up the face and looks great in a natural makeup look. You want to choose a shade that matches your natural flush of the cheek as this will flatter your skin's undertones. I recommend using a cream blush for the most flattering natural result but if you only have a powder blush then just make sure your foundation is set prior to applying your powder blush.

Use a large fluffy blusher brush if you are using a powder blush or use your fingers to apply a cream blush. Apply your choice of blush to the apple of the cheek and blend out towards the tops of the ears for a natural look.

Underpainting

Another great trick to try if you struggle with applying blush – maybe you apply too much, put it in the wrong place or you don't blend it enough – is a technique called underpainting. This is where you apply lots of your cream blusher to the apples of your cheeks or on your cheekbones before any foundation or concealer is applied. You then buff your foundation over the top, blending the blush in seamlessly for a natural flushed appearance that looks like it is coming from within, giving you a fresh, bright, youthful, natural looking complexion.

Bronzer

Bronzer is a great way to give yourself a natural glow. Lightly brush bronzer all over your face or along the cheekbones. If you don't like bronzer then just use your blush instead but don't use both. For the most flattering result, use a liquid bronzer or try adding a few drops of bronzer to your moisturiser for a healthy radiant looking finish for those clear skin days.

Highlighter

I recommend, when creating a natural look, using cream products and this goes for highlighter too, as unlike powders, the cream product blends and sinks into the skin giving you the fresh, radiant, lit from within glow.

If you choose to use highlighter, apply it to the tops of the cheekbones, bridge of the nose, cupid's bow and brow bone using a fan brush but remember to work with your face shape and highlight where needed to enhance your face.

Eyes

You can quite simply apply a couple of swipes of

mascara to your lashes and you would be good to go. But if you wanted to enhance the shape of your eye, you can choose to add eyeliner to your upper lash using a pencil to make your lashes look thicker and your eyes more defined. Apply the pencil line and smudge with a pencil crease brush or a fingertip. Don't bother creating any wings or flicks, just keep it soft and smudged and blend it into the roots of the upper lashes.

Apply a nude liner to the lower water line and inner corner to help make your eyes look bigger and more awake.

Natural makeup is all about flattering your features, so your eyeshadow should make the most of your eye shape. Neutrals like soft browns, beige, peach, and taupe work well with all eye colours. Using two shades, you can softly contour the eye to give definition by applying the darker shade into the crease and outer third of the eye and applying a lighter shade on the lid to add depth.

Brows

Brush through your brows with a clean spoolie brush

and fill in any gaps with a powder or pencil to softly define the brow to frame your face. A quick and simple trick to try is lift the arch of the brow and draw small strokes along the top edge of the brow for an instant brow lift.

Lips

Exfoliate your lips to remove any dead skin with a gentle lip scrub to make your lips look healthier, smoother and bring out their natural colour. Apply a moisturising lip balm or serum and let this sink in. Ensuring you prep your lips well before applying any other products will give you a blank smooth canvas to work on and will make your lip products last longer.

You can use a tinted lip balm, lipstick, gloss or tint, it is your choice with a natural makeup. I like to use a lip tint or balm in one shade darker than the natural lip tone to define and plump the lip. As it is a tint there is no extra texture applied to the lip so your natural lip can shine through. That being said, you can always line your lips and apply a lipstick, it is entirely up to you and depends on your desired natural look.

Easy Natural Look

1) Prep the skin and apply your primer.

2) Apply your skin tone liquid foundation to the face using fingers or a brush. Apply to the centre of the face and blend outwards towards the hairline, blend well down the neck.

3) Apply concealer to any blemishes and dark circles using a shade lighter for under the eye and the same shade of concealer for everywhere else. Apply with a fluffy brush and blend well.

4) Apply eye primer to the eyelid and set well.

5) Using a fluffy crease brush, dip just one side of the brush into a warm taupe-brown or an eyeshadow shade that is slightly darker than your skin tone. Pat this colour onto the outer corner of the eye using small circulator motions to blend. Blend the shadow into the socket of the eye and across towards the nose in a windscreen wiper motion (back and forth).

6) Using a flat shader brush, apply an eyeshadow

one to two shades lighter than your natural skin tone for an eye brightening effect. This can be matte or shimmer, it's your choice. Apply onto the eyelid and inner corner of the eye. You can even skip this step if you want to and just use the taupe shade in the crease for a bit of definition.

7) Apply brown or black liner to the upper waterline and lash line. Use a pencil crease or fingertip to blend and smudge slightly into the roots of the lashes for definition and to make the lashes look fuller and thicker. Apply a nude liner to the lower waterline to open up the eye.

8) Curl your lashes and apply mascara. I usually do my lashes after applying my base.

9) Set all your makeup with setting powder or spray.

10) This is an optional step - using a slightly darker foundation or contour powder, apply to the contour of your face with an angled contour brush, working with your face shape. You may not need to contour for a natural

makeup, it's up to you and depends on your desired look.

11) Apply a cream blush to the apple of the cheek, bridge of the nose and tip using fingers and blend out and up towards the top of the ear for a naturally lifting effect. Cream blush is brilliant to use on mature skin regardless of whether it's a natural look you are going for.

12) This is an optional step - apply your cream highlighter to your cheekbones, bridge of the nose, brow bone arch and cupid's bow.

13) Exfoliate your lips and apply your lip balm or tint that is one shade darker than your natural lip to your lips.

14) Fill in your brows with pencil or powder and softly define the brow.

Apply a setting spray to prolong your makeup to last you all day.

A Natural Smoky Look

1) Prep the skin and apply your primer.

2) Apply your skin tone liquid foundation to the face using fingers or a brush. Apply to the centre of the face and blend outwards towards the hairline. Blend well down the neck.

3) Apply concealer to any blemishes and dark circles using a shade lighter for under the eye and the same shade of concealer for everywhere else. Apply with a fluffy brush and blend well.

4) Apply eye primer to the eyelid and set well.

5) Draw a black or brown eyeliner pencil across your upper lash line, waterline and outer third of the lower lash line.

6) Blend with a pencil crease brush or fingertip into the roots of the lashes on the upper and lower lash lines.

7) Using a large fluffy crease brush, sweep a medium brown shade over the entire eyelid and into the crease and blend well.

8) Apply a dark brown eyeshadow into the crease to intensify with a fluffy crease brush for a softer application.

9) Using a light taupe neutral shade, blend

around the outer edges of the previous colours to act like a transition shade to help blend and soften further.

10) Apply mascara to the top and bottom lashes.

Apply setting spray to prolong the stay of your makeup.

Recommended Tools

Please see the Eye Makeup Brushes Section for my recommendation of brush shapes to use when creating all of your eye makeup looks.

Natural makeup looks are all about feeling like the best version of yourself. Ultimately there is no official definition of natural makeup so as long as you feel beautiful and confident, then go with it and enjoy the skin you are in.

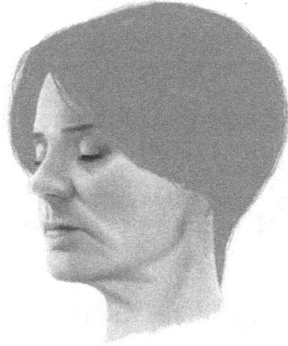

18. MATURE MAKEUP

Depending on age, skin type and undertones, each person's cosmetic needs are different. Mature skin has its own characteristics and needs that other skin does not.

I am here to tell you that regardless of your age, you should feel great about expressing yourself through makeup. I am going to give you lots of hints and tips that you can use to enhance your features and work with your mature skin to achieve its best results. As you age the skin's needs change and so should your makeup application. You will find eyeshadows and eyeliner will wear differently and your favourite colours may not quite sit right.

Foundation and Skin

Skin prep is important with any makeup but especially with a mature skin to help replenish its elasticity and smooth out any unwanted textures. Using a moisturiser that contains SPF all year round will help reduce the signs of sun damage and premature ageing of the skin.

Unfortunately, you can't hide wrinkles but you can help to smooth some of them out by staying hydrated and moisturised.

I recommend applying a moisturising eye cream to the eyelid and the undereye area to ensure this area is properly hydrated. Use a formula that is non-greasy. Ensure you prime your eyes along with the rest of your face for a smoother long-lasting application and apply a lip balm or lip plumper to your lips before applying any makeup products to make them fuller and more youthful.

When I am working with a mature client, I always like to warm up the makeup base by one to two shades to stop them looking too washed out and I recommend that you do the same. Apply your foundation to the centre of the face, where it's likely you need the most coverage and blend towards the ears, hairline and neck ensuring it is blended well below the jawline and down the neck to remove any harsh lines.

Choose a satin or dewy finish and liquid or cream formulas applied with a stipple or buffing brush for your most flattering natural result.

When applying your concealer to your under eye area, make sure you add it to the inner corner of the eye as this is often an area that appears darker as we age. Once you have applied your concealer and blended it in, let it sit on the skin for a couple of minutes so it soaks in before setting it with a light swipe of translucent powder.

You may find your makeup is not lasting as long as it used too so making sure you prep, prime and set your makeup is really going to help. However, don't go patting on that powder puff just yet. Instead, I recommend you use a moisturising setting spray to help keep your skin looking fresh and dewy all day.

Blush

I recommend using a warm cream blush or a gel over

powder as this is going to give you a beautiful natural flush to the face, giving it a natural, youthful glow. Instead of applying the blush to the apple of the cheek, apply blush to the top of your cheekbone nearest your ear and blend it in towards the centre of the face with a fluffy blush brush or a contour brush, this will help lift any face shape.

Whilst I like to use dewy or satin finishes for my clients with a mature skin, overly shimmery, glittery products are going to accentuate any texture you have in the skin, including pores, wrinkles, fine lines, acne and scarring. It can actually age you and highlight the skin's imperfections rather than just enhancing your features, so I would avoid shimmer finishes on a textured skin.

You can use a matte bronzer to warm up your complexion further by applying it to the cheekbones, jawline and nose for a sun-kissed youthful look.

Lipstick

Prep and prime your lips, and if they are particularly flaky then lightly exfoliate them before applying any products for a smoother application.

As we age, we lose elasticity in our skin causing wrinkles and fine lines to appear. This is especially prominent around the lips and this can cause a problem with lipstick products bleeding or slipping into those fine lines only to accentuate them more. Using a lipliner will combat this problem and define the lips, making them appear fuller and symmetrical.

When applying your lipliner use small strokes rather than trying to line the entire lip in one go. Use little feathery strokes or dashes to create your lip shape, apply an X onto the cupid's bow for definition and symmetry, and join them together. Apply your lipstick with a lip brush for a more precise application. Use a square-ended brush dipped into a translucent loose or pressed powder and apply this right along the edge of that lipliner to prevent any slippage of the liner or lipstick throughout the day.

To choose your suitable colour see the section on lipstick colours but I recommend working with your natural skin undertone, keeping to warm tones if you have warm skin or cool tones if you have cool skin. Although we are always trying to warm up a mature skin which goes for lips as well, as we lose a lot of colouration in our lips as we age causing them to appear paler. We want to be reintroducing that colour back into the skin for a natural look. Choose one to two shades darker than your natural lip colour for a more youthful pout.

Eye Makeup

As we age, our eyelids thin and become more transparent. This shows through more uneven skin tones like purples, blues and red tones. Before you apply any eye makeup products always make sure your eyelids are well primed and neutralised.

Apply a thin layer of eye primer and skin-toned concealer to the lids to neutralise and even out skin tones, giving you a blank canvas to work on that will boost your colours and prolong the durability of your makeup.

Applying an under eye primer before applying your concealer and foundation will help prevent the products from settling into the fine lines.

There is no one look that is suitable for a mature eye, this is all down to your taste and desired look. However, as we age, losing the elasticity in the skin can cause the eyelids to become loose and often become hooded causing you to slightly alter how you may have applied your shadows and eyeliner in the past.

Please see the Eye Shape Section to find looks that will suit your eye shape, including a smoky eye, but remember to use satin shades rather than shimmer or totally matte finishes as they both emphasise fine lines and texture. Satin cream eyeshadow works well on mature eyes; they are easy to apply and will sink into the skin giving luminosity without the shimmer. They often come in a variety of coverage ranging from sheer to opaque so you can choose which finish you like.

Use a nude pencil liner along the waterline to make your eyes appear bigger and more awake, and apply this same shade to the tear duct and inner corner of the eye to make your eyes appear brighter.

I don't recommend using a graphic liquid or gel liner for a mature eye as due to the nature of the thinning skin, it is likely to distort the finish. Instead, I would go for a soft pencil and apply this along the upper lash line in small dashes then use an eyeshadow applied on top and buffed into the lashes for a more natural result. Apply the same liner to the upper waterline to make the lashes appear fuller and add definition to your eye without it being too harsh.

I recommend using a small shader or eyeshadow brush and start with your eyeshadow on the outer corner. Blend this across the eye towards the nose, this is going to ensure that the colour gets lighter across the eye, making your eyes appear bigger.

Lashes

Curl your lashes before applying mascara to make your eyes look more open and bigger. I recommend using a mascara with a tubing formula to lengthen and thicken sparse lashes or you can get smudge proof formulas or mascaras that are designed to be used on the lower lash line.

Applying a setting powder along the lower lash line will help prevent your mascara and eyeliner from transferring and slipping down the face.

Brows

As we age, our brows tend to stop growing back after

waxing and over tweezing and often they start to lighten.

Let's keep things simple when it comes to doing your brows. Using a soft powder or brow pencil is all you're going to need. Be careful not to overdo your brows as you want the brow to frame the face and eyes but not to be the focal point of the face.

If you want to emphasise the arch of the brow, I recommend lifting the brow with an index finger from the forehead directly above the arch and concentrate your powder or pencil across the top of the brow in soft feathery strokes to replicate individual hairs to fill in any sparse areas, this will instantly lift the brow.

Use a matte highlight shade or light-toned concealer instead of a shimmery shade, applied under the brow arch to emphasise that lift.

I want you to feel confident and beautiful in expressing yourself through your makeup so you should use whatever products and techniques that you like. These are just guidelines to give you your most flattering results for your skin.

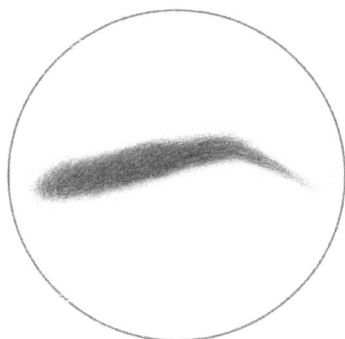

19. BROWS

BROW PRODUCTS

A brow frames the face, it is not supposed to be the focus of a face.

There are so many brow products available on the market, it's hard to know which type is the best. How do you even begin to choose? Is it ink, powder, pencil or pomade and what colours should I use? It's a minefield. Hopefully, I will be able to help shed some light and equip you with everything you need to know when choosing and applying a brow product that is perfect for your brows.

Let's look through the range of brow products.

Pomade

This is a fantastic product for someone with a thicker, longer brow and it will really help define a powerful brow. Use a light hand when applying pomade and start in the centre of the brow, working towards the tail in soft feather-like stokes. Pomade is the go-to product you see on social media so if you like that look then this is the product for you. You can use a spoolie brush to soften the edges.

Ink/Marker

This product looks like a felt tip pen or liquid eyeliner. It is a fantastic, versatile product that is great for covering scar tissue and gaps in the brows and is used to create the effect of individual brow hairs. When combined with a brow powder you can create a realistic brow even if you don't have any hair. This type of product needs to be used with a steady hand and a keen eye for detail. The ink brow products with a micro fine nip creates the effect of microblading your brows. It applies three ink strokes at a time and when built up creates the effect of precise individual growing brow hairs. This product is easy to use and is becoming more and more popular with the public and professionals alike.

Apply with short feather-like strokes in the direction of the natural hair growth towards the tail. Use upward and outward strokes for the inner corner of the brows. Brow powder can be applied on top to add dimension and depth to the brow once the ink has dried. I have one of these in my personal kit as it is so quick and easy to use. I can add in extra hairs where my brows are more sparse and I am good to go, knowing it is going to last me all day.

Pencil

Pencil has always been a firm favourite and has been around for a very long time for good reason. The pencil is very versatile, easy to use and comes in a variety of different colours, and almost every brand of makeup has their own variation of a brow pencil. Often a pencil is dual-ended, either with a sponge smudger, mascara wand (spoolie) or a highlight shader for the arch of the brow on the other end.

The pencil is great for creating soft, natural looking definition, filling in gaps in the brow and thickening a sparse tail of a brow. Always sharpen your pencil as a thin nib is great for creating realistic looking brow hairs when used in short feather-like strokes in the direction of the natural hair growth towards the tail. Use upward and outward strokes for the inner corner of the brows. The smudger can be used to blend and soften a harsh brow line, and a mascara wand is used to brush through the brow before and after applying your brow pencil.

Powder

This is another popular choice for any makeup kit and what's good about this product is you probably already own it, as any matte eyeshadow can be used as a brow powder. Just opt for natural, neutral colours like taupe, browns and khaki. Khaki is a great colour to use in your brows if you are a redhead.

Powder is applied using an angled thin brush and helps fill in any gaps or sparse areas. Powder gives a softer effect than many of the other brow products and is really easy to use and fix if applied too heavily.

Powder can be used to fix other brow products such as the pencil and creams. Make sure when using powder that you brush through the brows with a mascara wand to help soften the edges. Choose a colour that is close to your base hair colour, I tend to go for one shade lighter than my base to begin with as I often find it appears darker once applied and looks more natural.

Gel

This gel formula comes in various colours including clear. This product is an all-in-one, it adds colour and fullness and provides a subtle hold. It is used to tame an unruly or coarse brow.

Use this product sparingly. Remove extra product from the applicator then, using a light hand, backcomb your brow (against the hair growth direction) as this will apply the gel formula all the way around the brow hair and fluff them up making the brow appear fuller. Make sure to brush the brows back into the natural hair growth direction.

When it comes to filling in, colouring or defining your brow there are lots of products to choose from, just make sure you choose a formula/product that you like and that you are comfortable applying. If you think you require practice or you are perhaps too nervous to try, then opt to use the easier products like powder and pencil first and get used to defining and shaping your brow. Once you are more confident then try pomade, ink or a gel formula.

MEASURING AND SHAPING YOUR BROW

A well done brow can really make a makeup look.

Brows always need attention as part of a makeup application. How much attention it requires is defined by the brow itself as some are naturally desirable and may only require a tidy up and a bit of powder to define it. Some brows may be sparse, narrow, thin or even stop short, these types of brow may require more work.

Choosing flattering eyebrows is all about selecting a brow shape that will complement and balance out your unique face shape. Before we get into measuring the brow, I just want to identify the three key portions of your brow: the start, the arch, and the end or the tail, and discuss the terminology used to describe the shape and look of a brow.

The start refers to where the brow starts to grow nearest the bridge of the nose.

The arch refers to the curvature of the brow and how low or high the brow sits on the bone.

The end/tail refers to where the brow naturally finishes growing.

Arch Height

The arch height refers to how lifted the arch shape is and whether it's high, medium, shallow or straight.

Arch Shape

The arch shape refers to the pointedness of the peak of the brow arch.

Thickness

The thickness refers to the width of the brow and whether it's thick, medium or thin.

Definition

The definition refers to how the brow looks and whether it's soft, full or voluminous.

Length

The length refers to how far the brow extends. Is it:

- Normal - the brow tail extends only to the outer corner of the eye,
- Short - it stops growing before the end of the outer corner of the eye, or
- Extended - the tail extends past the outer corner of the eye.

Remember to always work with your natural shape by focusing on filling and shading with makeup. Removing hair should be a last resort.

There are some basic application techniques that all brow shapes use and there are some more specific techniques that are used for individual brow shapes, this section is about generic brow measuring and shaping.

Face shape plays a vital role when choosing your

ideal brow shape. To ensure your brows suit your face, you first need to think about your own face shape. Please refer to the chapter on face shape and find out how to define your brow to suit your face.

Application Techniques

- When working on a brow, you want to use upward strokes when applying your brow powder, gel or pencil as you don't want to flatten the brow. You want to accentuate the arch shape and its fullness. I always like to use a thin angled brush to apply my powders or gels, just make sure you remove any excess product from the brush first.
- Start from the ends of the brow and work towards the middle, so the darkest point is at the end of the brow and fade it towards the centre of the face near the bridge of the nose.
- Hair colour plays a major part in choosing your suitable brow shade. If you have dark hair and a light brow you may wish to darken your brow to match your hair.

- To create a more defined brow you need to brush (use a clean mascara wand) all the brow hairs straight up and trace the root line in a powder, gel or pencil. Brush all the hairs down and trace in the root line across the top of the brow, following your natural brow shape. Brush the hairs back into their natural position and fill in the centre using a natural colour focusing on the outer point and fading towards the centre of the face. If your frame lines are one to two shades darker than your brow fill colour this will accentuate the definition, just make sure you don't overdo the brow.

- You should not have to conceal around the entire brow to 'carve' out its shape. The brow shaping you did earlier will do this for you. You only need a little bit of highlighter under the arch and this will help your brows frame your face and not be the focal point of the face.

Your eyebrows are a built-in way to frame your

face and bring out your eyes. A defined brow can instantly make you look polished and put together.

Measuring Your Perfect Brow

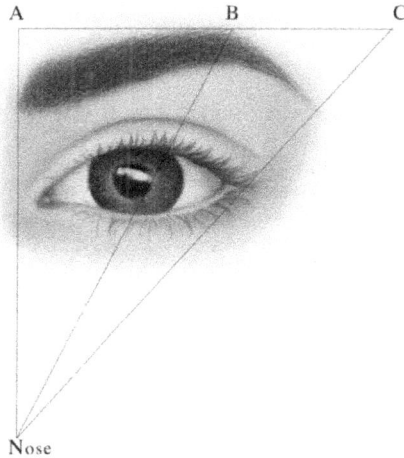

The three measurements used to measure a brow are all taken from the outer edge of the nostril. Use a straight edge like a pencil, pair of tweezers or makeup brush handle to take the measurements. If your nose is not perfectly proportioned then I recommend measuring the brow angles using your eyes as a guide instead. There are exceptions to this rule and you need to take your natural eye shape into consideration

357

too when creating your brow shape. For example, if you have wide-set eyes then you want to bring the brow further in towards the nose to create the illusion of closer set eyes, however on a normal or average set eye, having your brows too close together will create the effect of your eyes being too close together.

1) Using your chosen straight edge, place it on the outer edge of the nostril, as you see in the illustration, and point it straight up towards your hairline. This is where the brow should start, from the inner corner of the eye, ideally at a 90 degree angle. If your brow is sparse here then this is where you will need to fill in some individual hairs with your chosen brow product.

2) Looking straight ahead, use your straight edge from the outer edge of your nostril diagonally (22 degree angle) across your pupil and your brow. This is where your natural arch should be, just outside of this line. You want the arch to start close to the outer edge of the iris to prevent looking in a perpetual state of

surprise, however do not worry too much about the shape of your arch as your natural brow shape is the general shape you should follow to achieve a natural looking result.

3) Place the straight edge from the outer edge of the nostril diagonally at a 45 degree angle, making sure to cross the outer corner of the eye. This is where the tail of your brow should end. If the tail is considerably longer, then you might want to think about removing these hairs as this brow shape is likely to create the illusion of downturned eyes, or if you have hooded eyes then this will accentuate this further. If your brow is ever so slightly longer then don't bother with tweezers and just skip the brow filling at this part the brow and it will still look good. However, if your brow stops short then try applying light thin strokes in the direction of the hair growth to elongate the tail. I don't recommend applying a brow in one solid stroke as this can look overdone.

Who has time to measure and fill their brows every

day? Here is a great trick for speeding up your brow defining regime: lift your brow by placing your index finger above the centre of the brow, above the arch and lifting. Hold it in place and use feathery strokes with your brow pencil to draw in realistic looking brow hairs along the top edge of your brow, this will create the effect of a brow lift. Use a concealer to highlight the brow bone and voilà! Instant brow definition and lift.

CHOOSING YOUR PERFECT BROW COLOUR

When choosing your ideal brow colour, it is not always as simple as matching them to your hair colour. Sometimes lighter shades work better on a dark brow and vice versa, a dark tone can often look quite striking on certain shades of blonde.

Getting your brow shade wrong can really impact your entire look. That being said, you should wear whatever makes you feel confident.

- When choosing your most flattering brow

shade, you want to go about two or three
shades lighter than you think to prevent your
brows looking too overdone and odd.

- Try not to be too heavy-handed with your
  application and build up the colour slowly. It's
  easier to add than it is to take it away.
- Natural brows are not one block colour as
  some people would lead you to believe in
  their brow product selection.
- You can mix your own unique shade of brow
  powder by dipping your angled brush from
  one colour shadow to the next.

It is really important to think about the undertones
in your hair when choosing a suitable shade of
makeup for your brows.

Blondes

Blondes you are probably one of the hardest, besides
redheads, to choose brow shades for as it is all to do
with your undertones. Are you platinum, champagne
or ashy blonde? Cool blondes tend to suit grey, ashy
brown tones, sometimes even with a hint of khaki will

work well. If you are more of a strawberry, caramel or golden blonde, then you will want to use a warmer light brown taupe shade which works really well in those warmer undertones.

Redheads

If you are lucky enough to be blessed with auburn locks then, like the blondes, you want to look at your undertones as very few people truly have red brows. If you have light, strawberry blonde brows try a taupe, golden blonde shade. If your brows are warmer and more auburn then try an auburn shade.

There is so much choice out there now available for redheads, so go out and have some fun choosing your tone.

Brunettes

Dark hair doesn't necessarily mean you have to have super dark brows. The general rule for brunettes is to stay one or two shade ranges from your hair colour. If you've got ashy, cooler or light brown hair then a medium brown shade is going to work well for you.

I like to use an ashy mid-toned brown on dark

brows as I have found choosing rich shades to match the hair colour is often too warm for the brow.

Dark brows with darker skin tones look good when defined with a deeper dark brown tone.

The most flattering shade to use is one to two shades lighter than your natural brow/hair colour. My tip is to start off light and build up the intensity. It's always easier to add than it is to remove products, especially with the brows.

Rainbow

As well as the various brow products, formulas and natural shades available, there is now more choice than ever when it comes to colouring your brows, including bright neon and rainbow shades. This may be a little daring for some or perhaps it is the perfect addition to an already vibrant hair dye job or for someone who loves colourful makeup. You can go crazy creating endless looks with any colour brow that you wish with all the different formulas available.

BROW BRUSHES AND TOOLS

You want to choose a suitable tool when applying your brow products. Here are my recommended brushes that I like to use when defining and shaping a brow.

Brow Brush/Comb

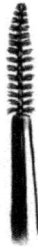

Also known as a spoolie, it looks like the end of a mascara wand. This is designed to comb through brows before applying brow products and can be used after to help soften and blend the brows. This tool can be used with any of the mentioned brow products.

Angled/Brow Brush

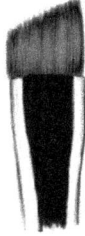

This is a great shape brush for precision work due to its thin wedge shape with dense short bristles, giving you total control of your brush strokes. Its angled shape is perfect for creating realistic looking brow hairs and is suitable to be used with powder, pomades and gels.

Square-ended Brush

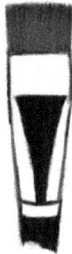

The square-ended brush is similar to the angled brush with densely packed short bristles but this brush has a straight edge rather than a slanted edge. The square-ended brush is a good shape for creating realistic brow hairs and is suitable to be used with all the brow products.

Slanted Tweezers

When defining and shaping the brow, it may sometimes be necessary to remove some stray hairs to help define the shape further. I recommend slanted tweezers or flat ended tweezers when plucking out hairs. Always make sure you stretch the skin when tweezing as this will help prevent accidently pinching your skin or tweezing too many hairs at once and ensure you pluck out the hairs with the brow hair growth. Do not overdo the plucking, do tiny bits and keep checking in a mirror.

Pencil Sharpener

If you are using brow pencils, don't forget to sharpen your pencil to create a sharp point for a precise application.

Warm up the pencil in the palm of your hand to soften the product for less drag and a blendable finish.

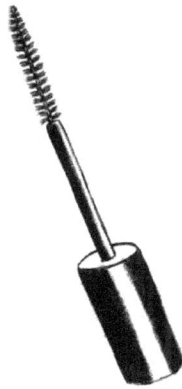

20. LASHES

MASCARA PRODUCT TYPES

There are lots of different types of mascara, some that boost volume and some that add definition or length. There are also various formulas including waterproof, growth enhancing, age reversing, moisturising and vegan friendly options.

Mascara is an essential item for any makeup kit as a swipe of this can really awaken the eye, bring definition and enhance the eye shape.

It works for both natural and dramatic looks and really finishes off a beautiful eye makeup.

There are seven main types of mascara for you to choose from and each one is formulated in a way to achieve a particular result; therefore it is important for you to choose the correct type to suit your eye lash needs. With so many different types, formulas and wands to choose from, that is easier said than done. I am going to help you choose the right mascara that is suitable for you.

Lash Lengthening/Fibre Mascara

This type of mascara is perfect for those with short or sparse lashes as this formula will extend the natural lashes. Lengthening mascara often contains small synthetic fibres that bind to the tips of the lashes, adding extra length and volume, causing the lashes to appear longer.

Tubing Mascara

Tubing mascara is designed to coat each and every individual lash hair like a tube, thickening the natural lash and adding extra length. This is an ideal formula for you if you have short or sparse lashes. This formula can be tricky to remove effectively so I highly recommend using micellar water which is made up of tiny balls of cleansing oil molecules suspended in water and is fantastic. It is my go to makeup remover and removes everything so easily there is no need for rubbing or scrubbing, this cleanser can also remove waterproof mascara.

Thickening/Volumising Mascara

A volumising mascara defines the eyes by making lashes appear darker and fuller, and is perfect if you have thin or sparse lashes. I recommend opting for a dark black mascara at least a few shades darker than your natural lashes for extra definition.

Curling Mascara

Curling or enhancing the curl of your eyelashes will make your eyes look bigger. Curling mascaras have a thicker consistency and a curved wand which helps the polymers in the formula curl the eyelashes. This is a good choice for someone with very straight lashes.

Waterproof/Smudge Proof Mascara

Waterproof mascara does exactly what it says on the

tin. No matter what life throws at your lashes, this formula is built to withstand everything including sweat, heat and water. This type of mascara is my go-to formula for my brides for when they shed those happy tears. It is rub resistant which can cause it to be tricky to remove without the correct eye makeup remover like micellar water. This formula can be quite drying on the lashes so make sure you remove all your mascara at the end of the day and avoid sleeping in it.

Non-clumping Mascara

You would think that a non-clumping effect would be a given when it comes to choosing your mascara, but you can actually get non-clumping formulas now.

This type of mascara gives the most natural look whilst still adding definition, but unlike the other formulas you may not be able to achieve as much length or volume from your lashes with this mascara.

Lash Defining Mascara

Lash defining mascaras are an all-in-one solution suitable for all lashes as this formula provides definition, volume, length and thickness and is even available in a waterproof finish. A good all-rounder to have in your makeup kit.

APPLICATION TECHNIQUES

You want to make sure you curl your eyelashes before applying your choice of mascara.

Look straight ahead and hold the lash curler open at the base of your eyelashes and press closed over your lashes (be careful not to pinch the skin). Now, look down and gently press the eyelash curler. Pump the curler a few times as you move up the lashes to the tips. A little neat trick is to heat up your eyelash curler with your hair dryer for a few seconds for a stronger curling effect (make sure you test the curler to ensure you don't burn or damage your skin and lashes).

1) Open your mascara and pull out the applicator. Wipe off the excess.
2) Look down, place your loaded mascara wand in the centre under your lashes and wiggle the

brush side to side whilst pushing upwards to coat every lash root to tip.

3) Use the mascara wand applicator's tip vertically for applying mascara to the corners of your eyes to ensure the lashes are coated evenly from base to tip. Using the tip of the wand will stop the transfer of mascara to the skin and will only be applied to the hairs for a more natural result.

4) Using a clean spoolie or clean mascara wand to brush the lashes through before the mascara has fully dried to remove and prevent any clumping.

Don't forget your bottom lashes, these tend to be shorter, finer and sparse when compared to the top lashes so require a softer hand and precise application to prevent smudging.

1) Wipe off any excess mascara from the wand and use the applicator tip vertically to coat

each lash hair without transferring mascara onto the skin.

2) Try tilting your head down and looking up to apply your mascara to your lower lashes.

How To Remove Mascara

1) Pour some of the eye makeup remover on a cotton pad.

2) Close your eyelids and rest the cotton pad on the top of your lashes for a few seconds, this will break down the mascara to ease removal.

3) Gently wipe the pad downwards, towards your lash tips. You can try putting a cotton pad underneath the lashes whilst you do this and this will help remove the mascara from the entire eyelash.

4) Repeat this process until all traces of the mascara are removed.

MASCARA COLOURS

Black

A universal rule is that everyone looks good in a black mascara even on the fairest of skin. It provides a dramatic frame for the eyes, so when in doubt just know that a black mascara should always be your first choice.

For very fair or red lashes, I recommend applying extra mascara right to the roots using a fine liner brush to help blend and define the entire lash length.

Brown

Brown mascara has become a lot more popular and suits all skin tones and eye colours. It is the perfect choice for the barely there makeup look. Make sure you choose dark, richer black-browns if you have an olive or medium skin tone.

Soft browns look great with blonde, light brown and light red hair, and for those extra fair eyelashes, this shade will make your lashes visible but still natural.

Blue

Blue can be a scary colour but it can look brilliant on grey-blue, brown or light green eyes. On fair skin this colour can really pop, but if you are a little shy of using blue, try applying a black mascara first then swipe on a couple of coats of blue after it has dried or go for a navy blue and this will brighten the whites of the eyes.

Purple

When I say purple, I don't mean neon unless that is your thing. I mean royal purple, plum and violet, these shades look fantastic with green, hazel and even blue eyes. If you have warm skin tones then choose a purple that has warm undertones, such as plum.

Darker skin or cool-toned skin look fantastic with purples that have blue undertones like violet.

Green

Green mascara, well I never I hear you cry. Green can complement any skin tone, just choose neutral tones for the rest of your eye makeup. If you are a little shy of the colour green then try applying your black mascara first then swipe a couple of coats of green onto the middle and ends of your lashes for a hint of colour.

Rainbow

There are lots of mascara colours available on the market so go crazy and have fun experimenting. Why not try a bold pink lash with pink brows, or how about applying some white lashes for a very avant-garde look. I absolutely love white lashes and love to utilise them for fashion shoots.

FALSE LASHES

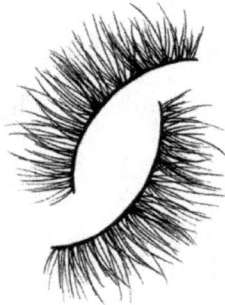

There are lots of different types of lashes from strips, cluster and individual lashes, and even magnetic varieties are now available. Much like the mascaras are formulated in a way to achieve specific results so too are false lashes.

They all have different qualities to enhance your eyes by providing length, volume, definition, glamour and drama.

False lashes come in a variety of styles, sizes and types and are made of different materials such as synthetic fibres, mink and even feathers, and you can achieve anything from a soft natural finish to a glam sweeping style.

Before choosing and using false lashes, it's important to know the differences in the various options available to find the perfect set of lashes for you.

There are three main types of false eyelashes; strip lashes, cluster lashes and individual lashes. These can be made of synthetic or organic materials, such as animal, human hair, paper and feathers.

Strip Lashes

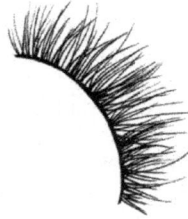

Strip lashes come in many styles to create different looks and are made from a variety of materials attached to a weft. The style you choose will depend on your eye shape, personal preference, budget and the look you are aiming to achieve, whether that be barely there and natural or something a little more glam.

Strip lashes offer a variety of sizes and finishes such as glamour, drama, lengthen, natural, volume and wispy varieties. The strip lash comes in four main types made from different materials including fur and human hair. The strip lash is versatile and can be trimmed to custom fit your eye shape.

Mink

Well known for their fluffy, soft texture, they are super lightweight and have a beautiful delicate curl.

This style of lash is perfect for adding volume, length and texture. The layering of the mink lashes provides a natural looking appearance. It's not the most humane and if you are looking for a more animal friendly version then you can get faux mink lashes that offer the same lightweight beautiful, layered texture but with a more affordable price tag.

Silk/Faux Silk

Another lightweight option for your lashes is the silk lash which gives a beautiful natural finish with a soft shine for a stunning enhancement. This style of lash is not as full or fluffy as the mink lashes but still beautiful and comfortable to wear too.

Human Hair

Many of the more subtle, everyday lash styles are made from human hair! These styles have lots of variety and multipack options so you can stock up on your favourites. These lashes provide a natural result whilst being comfortable to wear. They are easy to get hold of as they are available from most cosmetic stores and supermarkets and are an affordable option.

This is a great lash for beginners to practice their application with due to their flexible and thin band.

Synthetic

Synthetic lashes are the perfect lash if you want to create drama and glamour with your eyes, as this type of lash offers an extreme black finish with a thicker black band and shiny finish. I would not recommend this style of lash if you were looking for a more natural lash look.

Flare/Cluster Lashes (Bulb)

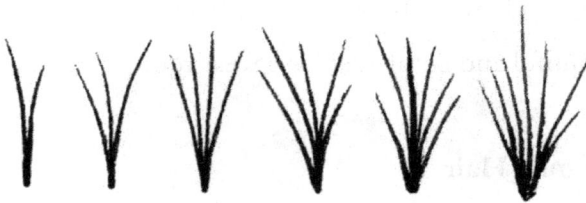

Individual flare lashes are a cluster of eyelashes attached to a tiny band called a bulb. These types of lashes are predominantly used by professionals due to the time-consuming nature of their application. As they are applied individually, they can be used to provide targeted application to fill in sparse areas and increase the lash fullness.

Flare lashes typically come in three different lengths and can be mixed and matched across the eye for a custom effect. These lashes can be layered to create a voluminous look, or you can just add a handful to the outer corner of the eye to create a flared lash effect that will help open up the eye.

This type of lash does require lots of practice to ensure that you get it right as it can really be obvious if incorrectly applied.

Individual Lashes

Individual lashes are used by professional lash technicians for eyelash extensions. This type of lash is more permanent and can last up to six weeks with infills. They must be applied by an expert hand because if they are applied incorrectly, it can be quite damaging for the lashes and, potentially, your eyes. The glue is very strong and you must have a patch test done 24 hours before having lash extensions. I thought they were worth mentioning as they are lashes, after all.

I love to have my lashes done for my holiday, as I

feel I can go makeup free with beautiful fluffy lashes and I just feel glam and confident all day.

Not all types of lashes will suit everybody's eyes as we all have different eye shapes and natural lash lengths. It is important to choose the right shape lash for your natural eye shape for a more coherent look.

I have provided a brief table to help you choose your ideal lash style that is suitable for your eye shape. To identify your eye shape please refer to the chapter about eye shapes.

Eye Shape	Strip Lash Style
Deep-set eye	Long and wispy
Round eyes	Criss-cross lashes
Mono lidded eyes	Multi-layered styles with long and short hairs
Close-set eye	Long, criss-cross lashes
Hooded eyes	Fluttery and long
Upturned eyes	Flared half lashes on the outer corner or criss-cross lashes
Almond eyes	Any type of lash is suitable
Downturned eyes	Flared lashes

Application Techniques For Applying Your Lashes

The weft band on a strip lash come in clear, white and black stripes. White strips are supposed to be invisible but if applied incorrectly can really show up if not camouflaged into the lash line. I normally opt for a black band as I find these the best to camouflage into the natural lash line and to blend with mascara and eyeliner, however the white strip or clear strip, if applied correctly, can look even more natural and great for an everyday makeup look.

1) Apply your chosen glue to the strip lash underside along the band edge and let the glue go tacky. This should take about 30-45 seconds. Bring your prepared, measured and cut lash up to your lash line and start from the inner corner ensuring some of your natural lashes are left so you are not gluing the strip lash right into the corner of the eye as this will likely be very uncomfortable. Make sure you glue the strip lash to the lashes and not the

eyelid skin as this will be uncomfortable to wear for a significant length of time.

2) Whilst looking down, place the pre-glued lash into the centre of the lash line and then press the lash into place from the inner and outer corner with tweezers or eyelash holders to press the lash on and ensure a tight seal. Once I feel it has dried, I do a tug test. Remove and reapply the lash if the edges have lifted at all as this will prolong their wear.

3) Make sure when applying your lash that you are applying the strip lash on top of the lash line. If you apply it from the side they may well stick but it won't look as good as applying them on top of the eye. You get a better curve this way and it is more suitable for any eye shape.

Application Tips For Applying Your Strip Lashes

- So many people forget this vital step! Make sure your lashes actually fit your natural lash line and eye shape exactly as this will ensure a more natural result and will be the most comfortable to wear too. Have you ever worn lashes and they have irritated the inside corner of your eye? Chances are they were too long for your eye shape or inappropriately applied to the lash line.

- Never pull your strip lash off the plastic backing, always use a pair of tweezers to lift and ease off an edge and peel away from the backing. This will prevent the lash from stretching, distorting and potentially tearing.

- The lashes need to be malleable and can be quite stiff from being in packaging so will require a stretch before being applied for a comfy fit. Hold the lash end with index finger and thumb on both hands then ripple the lash and shake it. This will help the fibres separate, creating a less rigid appearance on the eye.

- Normally you want your lashes to start after a few of your own lashes on the inner corner of the eye and you want the end of the false lash to end at your natural lash line to prevent the eye from looking droopy or heavy.

- When cutting your false lash always make sure you cut them from the outside edge and never from the inner corner as eyelashes are shaped for the eye so the lashes on the inside are shorter than the outside. If you cut the inside lashes your lashes will end up looking odd and the inner lashes will likely be too long and irritate your eye. Never cut the lashes themselves as the individual fibre is tapered into a point, like a natural lash, and if you were to cut them off they would end up looking blunt and fake on the eye.

- People may disagree on which colour glue is best. I personally use white as it dries clear. Sometimes if it's a little thick it can sometimes stay white but can be easily fixed with mascara and eyeliner. A black glue dries black and often shiny so it has to be applied perfectly with no lumps otherwise this will be visible on the lash line and can be hard to blend.

- Before applying lashes, I like to apply a little bit of mascara to the natural lash as I find it helps them blend a lot better. I then apply more mascara once the lashes have bonded to help the natural lash blend with the false lash.

- I try not to curl my lashes or my clients' lashes before applying the strip lash as I sometimes find it can become much trickier to apply the strip lash. But if you have particularly straight lashes then I definitely recommend curling those lashes before and even using a curling mascara before applying your chosen lash.

- Instead of fully closing your eye, try looking down into a mirror. This will stretch the eyelid and you will still be able to see as you can use both eyes.

- My favourite trick for blending in eyelashes is to get my clients to look to the outer corner of the eye and I run gel liner or pencil along the upper waterline in the inner corner of the eye up until the join of the strip lash. This helps the lashes really blend into that lash line. I even use this technique if my clients are not wearing strip lashes but I will run the eyeliner across the entire length of the upper waterline as this makes the natural lashes appear fuller and really does make a huge difference to an eye makeup.

How to Remove Lashes

An oil-based makeup remover can be used to remove most lash glues but most lash glues are gentle enough on the natural lash that the stripes can be gently peeled off without any damage being caused to the natural lash.

Lashes can be worn multiple times as long as they are cleaned between each wear to prevent the spread of any bugs and bacteria. Cleaning your lashes will also stop the lashes from becoming clogged with mascara and glue and looking spiky and unnatural when applied.

How to Clean Your Lashes

Put your strip lash onto a paper towel and spray with IPA or a brush cleaner to gently remove any glue or mascara residue with a cotton bud. Once clean, give your lashes a comb through with a mascara wand and leave them to dry. They are now ready to wear again.

Recommended Tools and Equipment

You want to choose suitable tools when applying your lashes. The following are my recommended tools that I like to use when applying, removing and cleaning my lashes.

You will need:

- Your chosen lash style suitable for your eye shape and desired look.
- Scissors - ideally small nail scissors for trimming your lashes to fit your natural eye shape and length.
- Lash glue - to adhere false lash to the lash line.
- Lash tweezers - for holding the lashes whilst applying the glue and for applying the strip lash to the lash line accurately.
- Lash curlers - to curl the natural lashes before applying your false lash.
- Eyeliner and eyeliner brush - for blending in the band into the lash line.
- IPA and cotton buds - to clean the lashes to

remove any glue, bacteria and mascara residue.

Magnetic Lashes

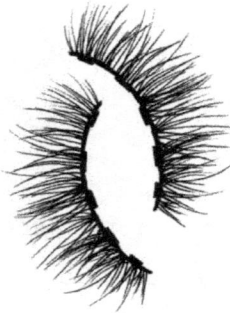

One of the best things about magnetic lashes is that they can be readjusted without any mess or reapplication of glue. You can just peel them off and reapply them resulting in a stress-free application as you won't end up ruining your beautiful eye makeup with glue and reapplying.

If you are fed up with trying to apply sticky lashes that ping off or do not fit, or perhaps you have never tried lashes before, then magnetic lashes could be perfect for you.

Magnetic lashes look and act like strip lashes but instead of gluing the weft band to your natural lash line these have tiny magnets along the band that attach to either eyeliner or other magnetic lashes. Let me explain.

There are two main types of magnetic lash. Both are magnetic but one style is made of two lashes that magnetise to each other and snap over the natural lash sandwiching your lashes between the false lashes for a secure fit.

The other type requires you to apply a magnetized eyeliner to your lash line first and then the lash magnetises to the eyeliner. This will require a steady hand to apply the black eyeliner so may require more practice.

You will still need to measure these lashes so that they fit and suit your eye shape as they often come on quite long weft bands and will require cutting. Be careful to ensure you only cut from the outer edge and try not to remove too many magnets otherwise they won't stick.

Application Techniques for Applying Your (Sandwich) Magnetic Lashes

A common problem found with both types of magnetic lashes is the edges tend to lift, so to combat this problem, I recommend cutting your magnetic lashes in half and applying each section separately. If it is the eyeliner system then you can swipe on your chosen eyeliner design, whether it's thick, thin, winged, etc, then apply your section of lash to the inner side of the lashes first. Then apply the outer lashes last. If the lashes make your eye appear droopy then you may still need to trim the weft of the lashes or try a different style that will help lift and open up the eye.

I found the sandwich magnetic lashes (two wefts of false lashes that magnetise to each other whilst sandwiching your lashes in between) difficult to apply using my fingers. I would recommend using the lash applicator that often comes with, or is available to purchase for use with, magnetic lashes.

1) Peel the upper lash from the backing.
2) Measure and using lash scissors, carefully trim the upper lash directly in half, ensuring you don't trim any of the magnets off the lash band unless you need a shorter weft.
3) Cut the lower lash into two and trim to the

same length weft as the top lash.

4) Position one half of the upper lash on top of your natural lashes close to the nose, making sure it is as close to your natural lash line as possible.

5) Position and apply one half of the lower lash underneath, sandwiching your natural lash between the upper and lower false lash, and they should click together.

6) Apply the other two outer halves. Repeat previous steps until you have applied both sets of lashes.

Application Technique Using a Lash Applicator

You still need to trim your lashes to fit your overall eye shape and length, and you can cut them in half if you will find it easier to apply. The difference being instead of using your hands, you use what looks like an eyelash curler to apply and clamp your lashes.

1) Put the top lash onto the top of the lash applicator making sure the eyelash strip faces your eye.

2) Put the bottom lash on the bottom of the lash applicator making sure that the eyelash is facing the same direction as the top lash.

3) Bring the applicator to your eye and whilst looking down or straight ahead, clamp the applicator closed on the lash line without pinching the skin, ensuring your natural lash is between the two magnetic lashes and press closed to seal the magnets together.

This sounds like an easy technique, but I found that the lashes can end up sticking to the applicator so you may have to practice a lot to master this technique.

Magnetic lashes are safe to use around your eyes but I don't recommend sleeping in them and you must make sure you remove them and any magnetised eyeliner before having an MRI Scan.

As always please follow the manufacturers guideline on every strip lash you use and make sure you carry out a patch test with your glue every time just to be super safe.

Do not share your eyelashes, if you do always make sure to use IPA before you re-wear them or better still, get a new pair as you don't want to end up with a nasty eye infection.

Always wash your hands before applying your lashes and try to use an applicator where possible. Always remove your lashes and mascara before you go to bed otherwise you risk getting an eye infection.

Fantasy Lashes

I absolutely love creating my own lashes. You can pretty much make eyelashes out of any materials, fabric, paper, card, feathers, beads, sequins and glitter, all sorts. You just need to make sure they are not too heavy for the eyelids and that your glue is strong enough to hold your creations in place.

I just love creating fantasy eyelashes for catwalk and editorial looks. If you use a false lash as your base then you can use the false lash band to glue to the skin and you can adhere other materials on top of the lashes like threads, paper stencils, thin feathers, etc. You can dip your lashes in any colour of paint or glue and then dip them in glitter for festive lashes.

When it comes to fantasy lashes, your imagination is your only restriction. Why not go wild and create lashes to match an outfit. You don't have to apply fantasy lashes to your natural lashes, you can apply them under the eye or to your cheekbones. You could even use them to create outrageous brows. Obviously these are not designed to be worn daily but are such great fun to design and make and, of course, wear.

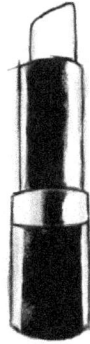

21. LIPS

TYPES OF LIPSTICK

There are many different types of lipstick available on the market and they all create different effects and characteristics.

You could have a different lipstick for every day of the week if you so wish, but with so many available on the market it is hard to decide what type, finish and colour would suit you best and it can be overwhelming to make a choice, it can also be costly if you get it wrong.

I am hopefully going to give you all the information you need so you can confidently choose the right type, finish and colour to suit you, your lips and your desired look.

The lipstick has been around for thousands of years and has been traced back to ancient civilisations when both men and women used to decorate their lips not only for medicinal purposes but also for aesthetic reasons too. Lipsticks were made from a whole host of ingredients including henna, fruits, insects, clay, rust and ground up jewels, and some that were in fact deadly, like lead. Luckily these days we don't use lead in our lipsticks, or any other harmful ingredients for that matter.

The Egyptians are considered to be the first ancient civilisation to love wearing lipstick as they have been depicted in hieroglyphics decorating their lips with lipstick shades from purple to black.

Whether you are looking for something subtle and nude, or you want to create a statement with a bright, or bold lip, lipstick is a quick and easy way to bring a look together, making any outfit fabulous and filling anyone with confidence and oozing sex appeal.

Prep and Prime

There is absolutely no point trying to apply a lipstick to an unprepped dry, chapped lip as your lipstick just won't last and it won't look good.

Make sure your lips are exfoliated and moisturised. I like to apply a balm to my lips and let it soak in whilst I do the rest of my makeup, then by the time I come to do the lips, they are ready for primer.

Lip primer works just like a facial primer, it prepares the lip for lipstick giving you a smooth canvas to work on and something for the lipstick to cling too, prolonging its staying power. If you don't have a lip primer then just make sure you apply a lip balm to the lip or use your facial primer on the lips before applying your favorite lippy for a smooth application.

Cream

Lipstick creams are soft and wet and often come in packaging with more than one shade of lipstick in them. Cream lipsticks come with a rose bud shaped applicator but can easily be applied using a finger for a softer result.

Lipliner/Pencil

Lipliner comes in the form of a pencil with lipstick inside. They are versatile, easy to use and can be sharpened into a point for precise application. Lipliner is used to line and define the lips, to help prevent your lipstick from bleeding, fill in any cracks in the lips, emphasise your cupid's bow and correct a lip shape or overline your lips to make them look fuller and bigger whilst increasing the longevity of your chosen lipstick applied on top.

I like to line my lips with my pencil and then I use it to fill them in too. Sometimes I will just use my liner as my lippy or I will apply a lipstick product or gloss over the top, depending on my mood.

Make sure you clean your pencil sharpener every so often with IPA (isopropyl alcohol or rubbing alcohol), to prevent it from harboring any germs and transferring them onto your lipliners and back onto your face causing breakouts and cold sores.

Liquid

Liquid lipstick is very similar to cream. It is a wet consistency, easy to apply and usually contains moisturising ingredients to prevent your lips from drying out. Liquid lipstick is often a gloss finish, but you can find liquids in a variety of colours and shades too. Liquid lipstick is often in a circular tube, like gloss and cream lipsticks but it also comes in a tube that you can squeeze directly onto your lips that looks a bit like a small toothpaste tube, with a sloped top to help spread the product.

Lipstick - Common

Lipstick is the bog standard. Everyone should be able to recognise the shape of a lipstick product, with its cylindrical packaging that is twisted from the bottom to push up the wedged shape of lippy from inside.

They are readily available across all makeup brands and come in a variety of different colours and finishes including gloss, moisturising, frosted and even metallic. If you want to discover more finishes then I discuss lipstick finishes at length in later on in this chapter.

This type of product is so easy to use and is swiped quite literally onto the lip. Make sure you do not twist the lipstick too high otherwise you may risk it snapping off. Another thing that is great about this product is if you use it a lot then it will morph to the shape of your lip for an even easier application.

Lipstick - Long Wear

Long wear lipsticks are designed to last four to eight hours so if you don't want the hassle of having to reapply your lipstick then I recommend choosing a long wear lipstick. Although it is long wear, if you plan on eating a meal wearing it then unfortunately you may still have reapply your lipstick as some oils in food will break down the pigments causing the lipstick to fade and rub off. If you want something more durable and long-lasting then I recommend you try a lip stain or tint.

Lip Stain/Tint

Lip stains and tints are brilliant for adding a wash of long-lasting colour, without adding any texture or shine to the lips, so they do not rub off but will fade over time. Lip stains come in a variety of colours and finishes from sheer and natural to vibrant and bold colours.

This product is very low maintenance, effortless, easy to use and versatile. It can be used as a cheek tint too, a handy bonus. Be aware, although stains are great, they can be quite drying on the lips so make sure your lips are well primed before applying a stain.

Lip Plumper

Lip plumpers work by irritating your lips to cause them to swell by bringing the blood to the surface of the lip. You can get different degrees of lip plumping, I even know of a product that you can literally turn up the intensity to achieve a fuller lip. I would not recommend using a lip plumper if you suffer with allergies or have sensitive skin, definitely do not use it if you have sore, chapped or dry lips as this will most likely not work but is likely to cause more issues and pain.

Crayon Lipstick

The crayon lipstick looks much like a lipliner but is chunky like a toddler's crayon. It is made up of a combination of lipstick and balm so it provides colour, shine and moisture to the lips and it also comes in a variety of finishes too. This product is really easy to use and you don't need to use it with another lip product, you can swipe these on and you are good to go.

Lip Balm

Lip balm is a must have in anyone's makeup kit and especially for someone who has dry or chapped lips. They are perfect to use all year round providing moisture to the lips in all weather. You can get lip balms that contain SPFs and some that are colour tinted to add that subtle hint of colour to your lips.

There is not always going to be one exact lip product that fixes all your lipstick troubles so don't be afraid to experiment and mix and match to find something that works for your lips, your makeup goals and your budget.

I am not going to tell you what product is best as it is all down to personal preference, suitability and the desired look you want to achieve with your lips, but hopefully I have given you lots of information, so you now can recognise the differences in lipstick types.

LIPSTICK FINISHES

There is a vast array of lipsticks products out there on the market. I want to explain to you the different types of finishes that are available and how to use them effectively, so you can make an informed decision on what finish you would like to achieve from your lippy.

Choosing your lipstick finish is all based on your own preference and your mood. Do you want something bold and bright, shimmery, glossy, perfect and matte, or do you want something you can meticulously apply in the morning and have it last all day, or would you prefer to swipe on your lippy on the go and be happy to replenish it through the day?

Matte

Matte lipstick is very popular at the moment and is a growing trend. This type of finish is very bold and usually a statement colour but it is hard to perfect due to its dry consistency. Some matte lipsticks can drag and emphasise fine lines and dryness of the lips so you must make sure the lips are well prepped by exfoliating and moisturising with a good lip balm before attempting to apply a matte lippy.

I like to create my own matte lipsticks by applying a cream-based lipstick to the lips and blotting with a piece of tissue, reapply for a more intense colour and then place one ply of tissue (separate a two ply tissue into its layers) onto the applied lipstick and use a power puff, sponge or brush to apply translucent powder through the tissue. The cream consistency allows for easier application with less drag and the powder gives that matte texture and finish and real staying power.

Satin

Satin lipstick gives a sheen like a cream lipstick but with the boldness of a matte finish. The added sheen provides moisture to the lips and prevents dragging and accentuating fine lines on the lips. It has a long wear time and comes in intense colours. I would recommend this finish for dry lips as it is more moisturising than matte or glittery finishes. Satin formulas often contain a high oil content so may appear darker in their packaging than when applied to the lips.

Cream

Cream is not really a finish but more of a consistency. The cream moisturises the lips making it easy to apply. It glides on with ease and is long wearing. They do tend to bleed so using a lipliner is a must. Ensure it is a complementary shade if you can't closely match it. A translucent powder applied to the edges of the lips will prevent the feathering without changing the colour of your lipstick like some lipliners can do once applied to the lips.

If you only have a different colour lipliner, ensure to coat the entire lip with the pencil and apply the lipstick over the top. This may affect the overall colour result but will look better than a miss-matched lip line or ending up with the 90's lip (a lighter lip colour with dark outer edges but it seems like this fashion may be coming back but with a more muted blend to emphasis the lips natural shape..

High Shine

High shine is a great alternative to sticky lip gloss. The lipstick is infused with a fine shimmer. This type of lipstick is hydrating and gives astronger coverage than a sheer lipstick but the shine fades over time so you will have to keep this lippy in your handbag as it does not have the staying power of matte or a cream lipstick.

Frosted

Frosted lipsticks seem to be making a comeback and are often applied on top of cream, satin or matte lipstick to add a frosted sheen. This type of finish is often pearly and can give an icy look to a lipstick. It can be quite drying due to the amount of shimmer, so you need to ensure lips are well prepped before applying this finish of lipstick as the shimmer can emphasise fine lines and wrinkles on the lips. I do not recommend this finish for mature lips. Once the colour fades, the shimmer can remain so use it sparingly.

Metallic/Glitter

Metallic lipsticks are highly pigmented like a matte lipstick but in a creamier consistency so allowing for a smoother application onto the lip. The colour is often toned with gold, silver or bronze reflective shimmer, a lot like a Ferrero Rocher wrapper. These finishes are not as glittery as frosted lipsticks but still give a lot of shine, like liquid metal. I would say these are more for fantasy colours rather than suitable for an everyday look but that is for you to decide.

Sheer

Sheer lipsticks give a subtle wash of colour to the lip, great for an everyday look that does not require much maintenance. The consistency is wetter so it is easier to glide on and does not sit in the fine lines, however it is not as long-lasting as a cream or a matte lipstick and will require reapplication.

The sheer finish is the most forgiving of lipsticks and is a great place to start if you want to start experimenting with your colour and then you can build from there. Sheer lipsticks like satin finishes have a high oil content so they can often appear darker on the packaging than on your lip.

Gloss

Lip gloss has a high shine that enhances the dimension of the lip and acts as a highlighter by making lips look plumper and bigger. I recommend using gloss if you have small or thin lips to enhance your lip shape and make your lips look fuller. Lip gloss can be applied on top of your traditional lipstick to add extra shine and dimension.

I recommend you try experimenting with the different types and finishes of lipstick and see what you like best. Have a go at making up your own custom colours or finishes. Mix together different types, try adding eyeshadow into a clear gloss. I had to do this for a shoot once as the photographer wanted a blue lip, so I mixed a vivid blue eyeshadow into a clear lip gloss until I was happy with the intensity of colour and it worked a treat, but due to its wetter texture it did not last as long as a cream or matte finish would have done. You can add eyeshadow directly to the lip and apply a gloss over the top. It is extremely drying on the lips so I don't recommend it for extended use but it is a fun technique to play with and you can create some fantastic fantasy colours without having to purchase multiple lipstick colours.

You should be able to choose the right type and finish for your lipstick that will suit you, your lips and your desired makeup look whether that be matte, metallic, cream, gloss or frosted. We now need to think about the colour of our lipstick – do we want something nude, neutral, natural or something bold and bright?

LIP COLOURS

There is so much choice when it comes to picking your lipstick products, there are palettes, glosses, stains, different finishes, frosted, metallic, matte, high shine and there is every colour of the rainbow available. How do you choose what is right for you?

I am going to give you some pointers to help you

confidently choose the best colours that are going to suit you, your skin tone and undertone.

There are so many different colours tones and hues of lipstick available that it can be a minefield when it comes to choosing your perfect lipstick colour. Even for me, when I am trying to find that perfect nude or brilliant red for my makeup kit.

All you need are some key guidelines and you will easily be able to choose a lipstick colour that is suitable for your skin tone and undertone.

What you need to remember is that we want to work with our skin's undertones.

By this part of the book you hopefully should know what the undertone of your skin is, however here is a little reminder for helping you find out if you have warm, cool or neutral toned skin.

Cool	Warm	Neutral
Pink, red, blue hues in the skin. Veins appear blue.	Yellow, golden, olive hues in the skin. Veins appear green.	Both pink and yellow hues in the skin. Veins appear green-blue.
Silver jewellery complements your skin.	Gold jewellery complements your skin.	Gold and silver jewellery both complement your skin.

It's important to note that skin tone and undertone are two very different things. Skin tone refers to the depth of your skin, e.g. the colour (fair, medium, tan and dark). Then there's the undertone which reflects the base tone of your skin (warm, cool or neutral). Someone with a fair skin can have warm undertones and likewise, someone with dark skin can have cool undertones, that's why it is so important to look at both the skin tone and undertone of the skin so you can choose the most flattering colour of lipstick to suit both.

Cool skin undertones look best in cool lipstick tones, warm skin undertones will look flattering in warm shades, and neutral undertones will look great in both warm and cool shades.

Skin Tone Common Colours

Fair:

- Light pinks
- Coral
- Peach
- Nude
- Dusty red

Medium:

- Rose
- Berry
- Cherry red
- Mauve

Tan:

- Coral

- Deep pink
- Bright red

Dark:

- Browns
- Plum
- Walnut
- Caramel
- Wine

Cool Undertone

The best lipstick colours for cool skin undertones have blue or purple base undertones (don't confuse base tone with an actual blue/purple lipstick). You want to choose a colour with the base tone of a blue or a purple, for example deep wine shades would have purple undertones, or cherry red has a blue undertone. But if you are looking for something more subtle and nude then you want to choose a shade that naturally enhances the natural colour of the inside of your lip, the darkest part with rosy, pinks and taupe-beiges like soft mocha.

Warm Undertone

The best lipstick colours for warm skin undertones have orange or red base undertones, think brick red, corals, oranges, golds and terracotta. If your skin is light then try using a paler nude and if your skin is dark or deep, try going for a richer nude with warm undertones.

Neutral Undertone

If you have neutral undertones then lucky you! This means you can pretty much wear whatever colour of lipstick that you please. Try using pink shades for fair skin, mauve looks great on a medium skin tone and try berry colours for deep and dark skins.

When it comes to choosing your perfect lipstick type, finish and colour then you should choose a lip colour that you feel most confident in. If you want to rock a matte red, go for it, if you want to wear a glossy nude then why not, have fun playing up your lips.

Tips on Applying Your Choice of Lipstick

- To test a lipstick in a shop, do not be tempted to apply it directly onto the lips. Just think of how many people will have done that, it is unhygienic and carries risk of infections. Instead, apply the lipstick to the tip of your finger as your fingertips are a closer colour to your lip than the back of your hand or wrist.

- If you're looking for a colour match close to your natural flushed lip colour then only apply it to the bottom lip, then you can compare it to the top lip. If it is drastically different then you may have to keep testing.

- I like to match my lipstick to the colour of the inside of my lip, the pinker wetter part, and no more than two shades darker than my natural lip colour so it still looks really natural.

- If you want your teeth to appear whiter then try using cool-toned reds. Avoid oranges at all cost if your teeth are not as white as you would hope, as this will only make them appear more yellow.

- If you want your lips to look bigger, without having to draw over them, try using lighter colours with glossy, shiny creamy finishes, as these will attract the light, making your lips appear plumper.

- If you have thin lips then I would advise not using matte shades as these will only accentuate the shape of the lip more.

- If you're using a bold colour but still want a natural finish; then apply your choice of lipstick to your bottom lip only and press your lips together and use a finger to pat the colour into the top lip. This will give a softer look. It's a good technique to use if you don't have the steadiest of hands.

- Apply lipliner first to prevent lipstick from bleeding. Apply your choice of lippy and tidy up edges with liner if needed or using a flat-ended brush to apply translucent powder right on the edges of the lips. This will help prevent your lipstick from bleeding but it will also tidy up any wobbly edges giving a lovely clean line, which can be further enhanced with concealer but make sure you blend it in and set it too. This works well with bold bright colours like reds.

- I not only apply lipliner to define a lip shape, I also use it to colour the lips before applying lipstick over the top as this gives it real staying power and I find it lasts much longer than when I apply just lipstick on its own.

- Sometimes, I like to apply the liner on its own or with a simple gloss applied on top.

Lipliner Colour

When it comes to choosing your lipliner to match your lipstick, try choosing a shade one to two shades lighter than your chosen lipstick colour to help with that seamless blend. Choose a lipliner shade that is in the same colour family as your chosen lipstick and ensure you match the undertone (cool, warm or neutral) and the overall colour choice.

If you use a lipliner that matches, or is as close as possible to your natural lip colour, then you will be able to use it with multiple lipstick colours, saving you money and the hassle of having to colour match each

419

and every lipstick that you own. You can even use this shade with red lipstick if you want a softer look.

I recommend using a red lipliner which either matches or is one shade darker for a beautiful defined look.

Tips on Applying Your Lipliner

- When applying liner to your lips make sure you fill in the entire lip as this will give your lipstick something to cling onto, causing it to last much longer.

- If you choose to use a lipliner that is darker than the lipstick, then make sure you blend it in towards the centre of the lip and apply your lipstick right to the edges. This will add lots of definition to the lips so make sure that they are even.

- Sharpen your liner before applying for accurate application. I recommend drawing it on the back of your hand first. This will round the very tip off the pencil so it is not sharp on the lip.

- If you find your lipliner is dragging, try rolling it in the palms of your hand to help loosen up the formula for a smoother application.

Reds

I love a red lipstick there is just something about it that screams confidence and oozes sex appeal. I believe anyone can pull off a red lipstick, it's just about choosing the right shade of red to suit your skin tone and undertone.

Generally warm skin tones work well with orangey reds, whilst cool skin tones suit reds with blue base tones.

If you want something bold and striking go for a matte red. If you are still a red virgin then opt instead to create a wash of red with a lippy mixed with a lip balm or a gloss, or use a moisturising lipstick as it is much sheerer. It will still be striking for you but will give you a margin of error so you don't have to feel guilty for applying it with your fingers. This will help ease you into wearing reds, then when you are feeling more confident you can intensify the colour.

A true red shade that has both orange and blue

undertones is going to look good on every skin tone because it does not counteract or contrast with any of the skin's undertones. I would recommend trying a true red if you want to be daring but are still a little nervous of colour choice.

If you are fair-skinned then you should look for a dusty, pinky red or coral shades. If you have cool undertones try using a raspberry colour and those with warm undertones should try reds with peach or orange undertones.

Tan and medium skin should look for bright reds, cherry and true reds, if you have cool undertones try wine colours or those with warm undertones should try orange-reds like corals.

Dark skin tones with cool undertones should look for rich warm reds and if you have warm undertones try metallic ruby reds or deep wine shades.

Tips on Applying Your Red Lipstick

- Don't forget to blot your red lipstick and reapply it for a more intense colour. Try using one ply tissue on the lips and pat a little translucent powder through to set the lipstick. Be aware this may mattify a glossy shade so you may want to apply a gloss over the top to add more shine.

- If you are using a traditional lipstick, you can also use a lip brush to apply the colour more precisely or use a finger for a softer diffused look.

- Are you scared of your red lippy transferring onto your teeth? Try sucking your finger after applying your lipstick, this will remove any lipstick from the inside of the lip and will prevent any transfer.

Red is an adventurous shade so be adventurous with your application. Wear whichever red makes you happy and wear it with confidence and you can't go wrong.

Nude

Like a red lipstick, I believe anyone can wear a nude lipstick. You just have to find the right shade that flatters your complexion. A nude lipstick should make you look fresh-faced, bright-eyed and not something resembling the living dead.

This happens when a nude tone is too light for the skin tone, as it will drain all the warmth and colour from the face ,making you pale and looking like a zombie.

To find your perfect nude lipstick you need to consider your skin tone, undertones and your natural lip colour. Look at your skin to see if you have cool bluish undertones or warm yellow undertones then choose a nude lipstick with the similar undertones to your skin, i.e. use warmer nude tones for a warmer complexion and use cool nude tones for a cooler complexion. We also need to take the natural colour of our lips into consideration too, when choosing the perfect nude shade.

Do you have naturally rosy lips? Then you are better off with using nudes with tones of rose.

Do your lips have a brown tint? Then make sure you choose a nude with a similar tone.

Do you have a lot of natural dark pigmentation in the lips? Then you want to choose a nude that is either identical or a shade lighter than your natural lip tone. Use a nude lipstick that has a hue of peach or even gold as the yellow undertones will neutralise the blue tones in the lips making them appear lighter.

Remember, we are not trying to erase our lips by using a nude so if you do end up choosing a shade that is a similar tone to your skin then you need to differentiate the lip colour to your skin tone by changing the texture. Use a creamier, glossier formula of lipstick, look for satin finish to give your lips a hint of shine or apply gloss to the centre of the lips for that kissable pout.

For light skin tones you should think pink. Choose nudes with a hue of pink like dusty baby pink or rose. It should still be soft, anything too beige will wash out your complexion, try using a rosy-beige instead. Using a sheerer formula, something with a little added shine will give the lips more definition and plumpness, and will stop them from looking too pale.

For olive skin, try using nudes with warmer undertones similar to your natural undertones. Avoid nudes that are lighter than your natural skin tone as these may result in you looking like you are wearing concealer on your lips. If you have light olive skin try using a light warm pink or warm beige. Make sure that it is distinguishable from your skin for the most flattering look.

If you have warm olive skin try using glossy caramel nudes and beiges that are darker than your skin tone to warm up your complexion.

Those with medium skin or tan skin should go for nudes with peachy undertones, salmon can also be a great colour to use. Try going for a golden beige that is slightly darker than your skin tone to give your lips definition.

For sun-kissed tanned skin, whether it's real or fake, use a glossy, shimmery nude to play up the sun-kissed glow of the skin. Try picking a glossy, shimmery bronze shade lighter than your skin tone to brighten the face for a more natural looking result.

Dark skin tones look fantastic with milk or dark chocolate nude shades, look for shades with berry undertones or even bronze or gold undertones with a shimmery, frosted finish for that kissable pout. Don't be afraid to pick up shades that match your skin tone or are a little darker, as lighter tones will likely look ashy against your skin.

Tips on Applying Your Nude Lipstick

- Pick nude shades darker than your skin to help define your lips.

- Try matching the nude tone to the colour on the outer edge of the lip as this is often darker than the rest of the lip, particularly if you have a darker skin tone.

- Try making your own custom nude by mixing colours together. Try applying a pencil to the lips and then applying your rosy nude over the top, or for a dark nude use a brown pencil then apply a beige-brown, rosy lipstick over the top and make sure you bend them together well.

- Use creamy, shimmery, glossy finishes of nude lipsticks to stop you looking like you are wearing concealer on your lips or apply a lip gloss to the middle part of your lips for that kissable pout.

- If you have blue eyes, try using cooler tones to play them up and if you have brown eyes, give warmer nudes with beige-reddish undertones a try.

Now that you know how to pick your perfect nude, it is also important to know how to wear it. What I love about nudes is you can literally wear them for any occasion, just remember to balance out your makeup when wearing a nude lipstick. If you have a dark smoky eye then go for a glossy nude, if you use a light nude shade on a pale skin tone, don't forget to play up that blusher to prevent the face from looking washed out and flat. I would advise not overdoing the nude/neutral makeup with light eyes and light lips as you may end up losing the definition of your facial features. Instead, try to play up your eyes, use layers of mascara, wear a natural smoky eye, by all means apply a neutral, natural eye but have a bold eyeliner, wear those faux lashes. Remember to define your facial structure too.

Have fun finding your perfect nude and remember, whatever you feel confident and beautiful in, go with it. There is nothing more beautiful than confidence.

LIP BRUSHES AND TOOLS

It is pretty easy to choose your lip brushes as most of the brush shapes used for applying lipstick are actually called lip brushes, so you can't go too far wrong by using one of these on the lips.

When working on lips, I like to use brushes that have short dense bristles to give me maximum control and finesse when applying my choice of lip product. I have listed my favourites below.

Square-ended Brush

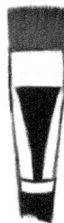

I use this brush shape when applying my lipstick. If I am not using lipliner then I like to use this brush to line my lips with the lipstick as this gives me nice control due to its shorter dense bristles. Then I use a rounded lip brush to apply the lipstick colour to the lips. I use the square-ended brush to neaten up any edges, that may not be quite perfect, with translucent powder. This is a great brush shape to have in your kit.

Lip Brush

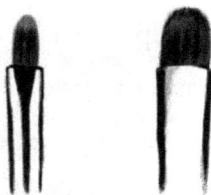

It does exactly what it says on the tin, however you can get different shaped lip brushes such as flat, tapered and rounded. They are all used to apply your lipstick, gloss, balm and lipliner if you don't have a pencil liner.

I really detest a lip brush with long thin bristles as it's near impossible to control and be precise with it, and when it comes to lips, especially if you are going for a strong lip look, you need to be precise with the application.

Pencil Sharpener

If you are using lipliner or eyeliner pencil then you

will definitely need a pencil sharpener to sharpen your liner into a nice point for accurate application. Don't forget to clean your sharpener once a month to prevent any build-up of germs from accumulating.

Lipliner

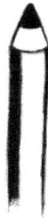

Although this is more of a product than a tool, I feel it is a really important tool to use for any lipstick application as it can really make a big difference to the overall look of the lipstick application and the longevity of the product. It is especially important when applying lipstick to mature skin or if you are trying to correct or alter a lip shape. Don't forget to rub the pencil between your palms to help soften the lipliner for less drag and an easier smoother application.

LIP SHAPES

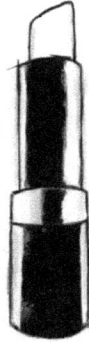

Lip makeup is a vital part of a makeup regime and it can really make or break your look. Whether you are going for a neutral nude or a daring red you need to take your natural lip shape into consideration.

If you want to change your natural lip shape then I recommend experimenting with various shades, finishes and colors of lipstick, and if you refer to the makeup tips below then hopefully these will give you some helpful tips on making the right choices with a lipstick suitable for your lip shape.

There are so many different types of lips. Some of us are blessed with fuller lips whilst others have thin lips, Lipstick has the power to make them appear more beautiful and enhanced. I have concentrated on the eight most common lip shapes as there are so many names and terms for different lip types, such as a lip bite and even the Coke lip! I wanted to use terms that I think will be more universally recognisable with the hopes that you will be able to identify the common characteristics within your own lip shape.

Thin Lip

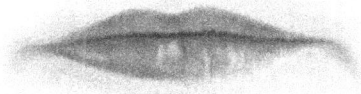

If both your upper and lower lips are thin, then you are considered to have a thin lip rather than a bottom or top-heavy lip.

I would recommend that you avoid using dark and bright lipstick colours as they will only make thin lips appear thinner. With that being said, I absolutely love a dark lip on any lip shape but if you are trying to change the shape of your lip to appear bigger then try applying glossy, creamy lipsticks in lighter shades to give the appearance of bigger lips.

Application Tips for Thin Lips

- Try overlining your lips with a lipliner the same colour as your choice of lipstick or your natural lip tone to make them appear slightly bigger, but don't overdo the overlining as you could end up with an unnatural looking pout.
- Shimmery, frosty formulas work well for thin lips as it adds volume and an enhancing effect.
- Try using a lip plumper or create the illusion by applying one colour of lipstick over the entire lip and then using a white or cream eyeliner or shimmery highlight onto the centre of the lip for a lip plumping effect.

Top-heavy Lip

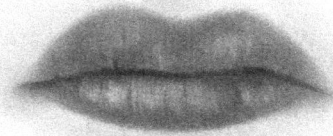

This lip shape is heavier on the top lip and tends to not have a pronounced cupid's bow.

The idea to 'correct' or change this lip shape is to balance out the bottom lip. This can be achieved by applying a slightly lighter shade of lipstick to the bottom lip than the top.

Application Tips for Top-Heavy Lips

- You can use a lipliner around the edge of your lips, following its natural shape on the top lip and then extend the bottom lip, lining the outer edge of the lip or even over draw it depending on the size of your lips. This will make your lips appear fuller and more even. You can use a lipliner or line your lips using a thin brush and your choice of lipstick.
- To make your upper lip appear slightly smaller, use a dark lip colour on it and go a shade lighter on your lower lip to even out your lips.
- If you don't want the faff of having to find lipsticks of similar colours then try using a

white or cream eyeliner pencil applied to the
centre of your lower lip to add a highlight and
thus making the bottom lip look bigger, this
will balance out your lips.

Bottom Heavy Lip

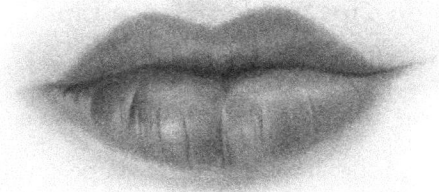

This lip shape is heavier and fuller on the bottom lip
so to correct or change this shape you need to add
more fullness to the upper lip. As with the top-heavy
lip shape, I recommend using that white or cream
liner but instead of applying it to the bottom lip, you
want to apply it to the centre of the upper lip instead
to add highlight and plumpness to the lip to balance
with the heavier bottom lip.

Application Tips for Bottom Heavy Lips

- You can use a lipliner around the edge of your lips, following its natural shape on the bottom lip and then extend the upper lip lining on the outer edge of the lip or even overdraw it depending on the size of your lips. This will make your lips appear fuller and more even. You can use a lipliner or line your lips using a thin brush and your choice of lipstick.

- To make your bottom lip appear slightly smaller, use a dark lip colour on it and go a shade lighter on your upper lip to even out your lips.

- If you don't want the faff of having to find lipsticks of similar colours then try using a white or cream eyeliner pencil, nude tone lipstick or eyeshadow applied to the centre of your upper lip to add a highlight and thus making the upper lip look bigger, this will balance out your lips.

Downturned Lip

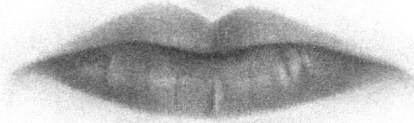

A downturned lip can often be found within other lip shapes, for example you can have a thin downturned lip, so it is important to identify the overall lip shape and then use appropriate techniques to correct the shape.

The aim is to provide lift to the outer corners of a downturned lip. I recommend using lipstick sparingly in the corner of the lips.

Application Tips for Downturned Lips

I personally have a naturally downturned lip shape and I will apply my favourite lippy and then actually wipe the corners off with my finger. Although it is not a very professional technique; it works for me and my lips. I find if I line the entire lip that I can end up looking sad or angry..

Full Lip

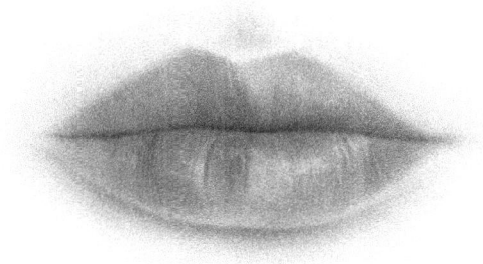

A plump, full lip is often protruding with a fuller bottom lip. I would love to have a fuller lip so I could do lots of different lip looks and colours. I personally say go for it and have fun with it, make the most out of your pout. But if you did want to make them appear slightly smaller, then it is probably best to avoid light, glossy, over glittery colours of lipstick as these will likely enhance the shape. If you are trying to make a full lip look smaller, you can use a nude lipstick that blends into the skin and this will help camouflage the edges of the lips into the skin, making them appear smaller. Try to use a darker colour lipstick as the dark tone will make a larger lip appear smaller.

Application Tips for Full Lips

- In order to draw attention away from your lips, play up your eye makeup. Why not try pairing a smoky eye with a nude lip.

- Highlighting your cheeks can also be a happy distraction and will make your face appear more balanced with a fuller lip.

- When lining a full lip shape, ensure to line inside the natural lip line as this will help the lip appear smaller and thinner.

Small Lip

This lip shape is not usually thin or wide, it tends to be full and protruding but of a smaller proportion to the full lip. I recommend using glossy, glittery textures with this lip shape to make the lips look bigger, and avoid darker colours as these will make your lips appear smaller.

Application Tips for Small Lips

- Brighter, soft shades usually look best on smaller lips and will brighten the entire face.
- Line your entire lip all the way round and blend to create a diffused soft edge, this will create a plumping effect and will lengthen the lip too.
- Apply a little bit of your makeup highlighter to your cupid's bow and the centre of your bottom lip to give the illusion of plumper, bigger lip.
- Light glossy pinks can make your lips appear thicker and fuller.

Uneven Lip

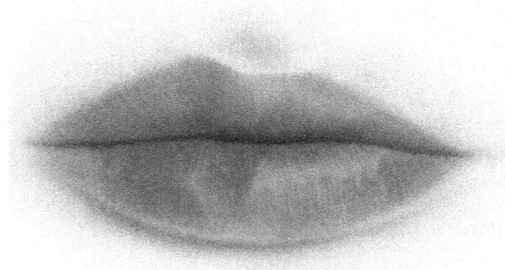

If your upper and lower lip do not match then you most likely have uneven lips. The aim here is to balance out the shape by ensuring the lips are of the same thickness. An uneven lip shape may also mean that the upper or lower lip is uneven across the width so you may have to draw your lipliner irregularly in order to create a symmetrical lip.

Application Tips for Uneven Lips

- Application techniques for an uneven lip are similar, if not the same, for a bottom or top-heavy lip. You use light tones on the thinner lip and darker tones on the thicker lip as this will help balance out the lip shape.
- I recommend doing one lip at a time. Start

442

from the top and outline your lip, making sure both sides are even, this may require you to overdraw part of the lip to ensure they are symmetrical. Then move onto the bottom lip. Make sure you blend your liner into the lip for a more natural result.

Flat Lip

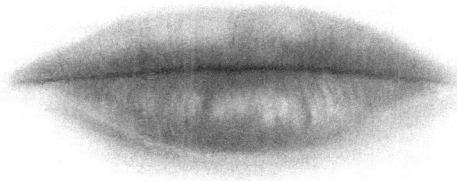

Flat lips tend to not have much dimension or depth so require dimension to be added by using light soft pearly, shimmery, glossy colours. It is best not to use dark or matte colours as these will only make the lip look flatter and smaller.

Application Tips for Flat Lips

- Ombre lip effects can work really well on this lip shape to add dimension. Try applying a

darker lipliner or lipstick to the outer corners
of the mouth and blend in towards the centre
of the mouth, then fill in the lips with a soft
or bright coloured lipstick within the same
colour family for an ombre effect.

- Apply the same colour lipstick on both lips
and then use a gloss or shimmer highlighter
applied to the centre of the lips for a lip
plumping appearance.

Application Techniques for Other Lip Shapes

- If your lips extend across your face to your
ears when you smile then you are considered
to have wide lips. If you want to correct this
lip shape then try overlining the lips towards
the centre of the lip to add thickness and
weight, therefore minimising their width.
- A heart-shaped lip will have the characteristics
of a prominent cupid's bow, often with a
heavy bottom lip. If you apply the same
colour lipstick on both lips and then use a
white or cream pencil or a lighter shade of

lipstick applied to the centre of the lips, this will enhance them and make them appear fuller.

Every lip shape is beautiful and I am a big believer in working with what you have got. You don't have to over draw your lips or only use nude colours, they are your lips and whatever you feel confident in will be beautiful.

You now have everything you need to make up your face!

I hope you have enjoyed your journey exploring makeup, face shapes, makeup techniques; in essence everything you need to know to confidently wear your makeup and feel good. Remember to experiment, try new techniques and most importantly – have fun!

ABOUT THE AUTHOR

Heather is the owner of Heather Card Makeup Artistry, a makeup service provider in Bristol and the South West specialising in airbrush makeup and providing personalised makeup lessons.

Heather is a professional makeup artist with qualifications and experience in teaching, and has over 10 years of experience working in colleges teaching various levels of media makeup across the South West. She has designed, developed and run qualifications, short courses and workshops ranging from VRQ's, NVQ's, BTECs and she was Programme Manager for a Higher National Diploma for 5 years before developing aspects for a BA Hons Programme.

Working closely with the NHS and Police, Heather has also developed and delivered workshops, providing training opportunities for cadets and NHS staff to learn to respond to A and E scenarios where she was in charge of producing realistic specialist makeup effects like pallor, bruising, burns, lacerations and open wounds.

Heather is currently working and living in Bristol, providing her airbrush makeup services to brides and clients for weddings and special occasions. She also provides tailored, personal makeup lessons to private clients in the comfort of their own home teaching them how to apply their own makeup.

Make Up Your Face was originally developed as an 8 page handout and has now grown to over 400 pages covering all aspects of makeup application, with the aim of making makeup accessible and personal to suit you and your skin.

If you would like to work with Heather, please get in touch via www.heathercard-makeup.co.uk or drop her a message on social media: @heathercardmakeup.

Thank you to the very talented Rachel for providing the beautiful illustrations for this book. If you would like to work with Rachel then get in touch with her via https://www.artistrachelcard.com or social media @artistrachelcard on Facebook and @rachelcardart on Twitter and Instagram.